Update on Surgical and Endoscopic Management of Emphysema

Guest Editor

CLIFF K. CHOONG, MBBS, FRACS, FRCS

THORACIC SURGERY CLINICS

www.thoracic.theclinics.com

Consulting Editor
MARK K. FERGUSON, MD

May 2009 • Volume 19 • Number 2

SAUNDERS an imprint of ELSEVIER, Inc.

W.B. SAUNDERS COMPANY
A Division of Elsevier Inc.

1600 John F. Kennedy Boulevard • Suite 1800 • Philadelphia, Pennsylvania 19103-2899

http://www.theclinics.com

THORACIC SURGERY CLINICS Volume 19, Number 2
May 2009 ISSN 1547-4127, ISBN-13: 978-1-4377-0552-2, ISBN-10: 1-4377-0552-9

Editor: Catherine Bewick
Developmental Editor: Donald Mumford

Thoracic Surgery Clinics (ISSN 1547-4127) is published quarterly by Elsevier Inc., 360 Park Avenue South, New York, NY 10010-1710. Months of publication are February, May, August, and November. Business and editorial offices: 1600 John F. Kennedy Boulevard, Suite 1800, Philadelphia, PA 19103-2899. Customer service office: 11830 Westline Industrial Drive, St. Louis, MO 63146. Periodicals postage paid at New York, NY, and additional mailing offices. Subscription prices are $242.00 per year (US individuals), $360.00 per year (US institutions), $121.00 per year (US students), $309.00 per year (Canadian individuals), $455.00 per year (Canadian institutions), $165.00 per year (Canadian and foreign students), $329.00 per year (foreign individuals), and $455.00 per year (foreign institutions). Foreign air speed delivery is included in all *Clinics'* subscription prices. All prices are subject to change without notice. **POSTMASTER:** Send address changes to *Thoracic Surgery Clinics*, Elsevier Journals Customer Service, 11830 Westline Industrial Drive, St. Louis, MO 63146. **Customer Service: 1-800-654-2452 (US and Canada). From outside of the US and Canada, call 1-314-453-7041. Fax: 1-314-453-5170. For print support, e-mail: JournalsCustomerService-usa@elsevier.com. For online support, e-mail: JournalsOnlineSupport-usa@elsevier.com.**

Reprints. For copies of 100 or more, of articles in this publication, please contact Commercial Rights Department, Elsevier Inc., 360 Park Avenue South, New York, NY 10010-1710. Tel: (212) 633-3812; Fax: (212) 462-1935; E-mail: reprints@elsevier.com.

Thoracic Surgery Clinics is covered in *MEDLINE/PubMed (Index Medicus)* and *EMBASE/Excerpta Medica*.

Printed and bound by CPI Group (UK) Ltd, Croydon, CR0 4YY

Transferred to Digital Print 2012

Contributors

CONSULTING EDITOR

MARK K. FERGUSON, MD
Professor of Surgery, Section of Cardiac and
Thoracic Surgery, The University of Chicago,
Chicago, Illinois

GUEST EDITOR

CLIFF K. CHOONG, MBBS, FRACS, FRCS
Associate Professor, Department of Surgery,
Monash Medical Centre, Monash University,
Melbourne, Victoria, Australia; Former
University Lecturer and Consultant
Cardiothoracic Surgeon, Papworth Hospital
NHS Foundation Trust; and Department of
Surgery, University of Cambridge, Cambridge,
United Kingdom

AUTHORS

FEREIDOUN ABTIN, MD
Assistant Professor, Department of Radiology,
Thoracic Imaging Research Group, David
Geffen School of Medicine at University
of California Los Angeles, Los Angeles,
California

KONRAD E. BLOCH, MD
Professor, Pulmonary Division, Department of
Internal Medicine, University Hospital of Zurich,
Zurich, Switzerland

CHRIS T. BOLLIGER, MD
Department of Medicine; and Tygerberg
Hospital, University of Stellenbosch, Cape
Town, South Africa

PAULO F.G. CARDOSO, MD, PhD
Professor of Surgery, Department of Surgery,
Division of Thoracic Surgery, Santa Casa de
Porto Alegre-Pavilhao Pereira Filho Hospital,
Universidade Federal de Ciencias de Saude,
Porto Alegre, Brazil

STEPHEN D. CASSIVI, MD, MSc, FRCSC
Associate Professor of Surgery, Division of
General Thoracic Surgery' and Surgical
Director of Lung Transplantation,
William J. von Liebig Transplant Center,
Mayo Clinics, Rochester, Minnesota

ROBERT J. CERFOLIO, MD
Chief, Department of Surgery, Division of
Thoracic Surgery; and Professor of Surgery,
Division of Cardiothoracic Surgery, University
of Alabama at Birmingham, Birmingham,
Alabama

CLIFF K. CHOONG, MBBS, FRACS, FRCS
Associate Professor, Department of Surgery,
Monash Medical Centre, Monash University,
Melbourne, Victoria, Australia; Former
University Lecturer and Consultant
Cardiothoracic Surgeon, Papworth Hospital
NHS Foundation Trust; and Department of
Surgery, University of Cambridge, Cambridge,
United Kingdom

GIORGIO F. COLONI, MD
Université di Roma "La Sapienza," Cattedra di
Chirurgia Toracica, Policlinico Umberto I,
Rome Italy

JOEL D. COOPER, MD
Professor of Surgery and Chief, Division of
Thoracic Surgery, Hospital of the University
of Pennsylvania, Philadelphia, Pennsylvania

MARCELO CYPEL, MD
Toronto Lung Transplant Program, Toronto
General Hospital, Toronto, Ontario, Canada

MALCOLM M. DeCAMP, MD
Chief, Division of Cardiothoracic Surgery;
and Visiting Associate Professor of Surgery,
Harvard Medical School, Beth Israel
Deaconess Medical Center, Boston,
Massachusetts

CHADRICK E. DENLINGER, MD
Cardiothoracic Surgery Resident, Department
of Surgery, Washington University School of
Medicine, Saint Louis, Missouri

JAMES M. DONAHUE, MD
Assistant Professor of Surgery, Division of
General Thoracic Surgery, University of
Maryland, Baltimore, Maryland

MELANIE A. EDWARDS, MD
Assistant Professor of Surgery, Division of
Cardiothoracic Surgery, Louisiana State
University, New Orleans, Louisiana

JONATHAN S. GOLDIN, MD, PhD
Professor of Radiology and Vice Chairman,
Department of Radiology, Thoracic Imaging
Research Group, David Geffen School of
Medicine at University of California Los
Angeles, Los Angeles, California

XAVIER GONZALEZ, MD
School of Medicine, University of Washington,
Seattle; and Spiration Inc., Redmond,
Washington

STEPHEN HAZELRIGG, MD
Professor and Chief, Division of Cardiothoracic
Surgery, Department of Surgery, Southern
Illinois University, Springfield, Illinois

SAMUEL V. KEMP, MBBS, MRCP
Clinical Research Fellow, Department
of Respiratory Medicine, Royal Brompton
Hospital, London, United Kingdom

SHAF KESHAVJEE, MD
Director, Toronto Lung Transplant Program,
Toronto General Hospital, Toronto, Ontario,
Canada

BALAKRISHNAN MAHESH, MBBS, MD
Surgical Registrar, Papworth Hospital NHS
Foundation Trust, Cambridge, United Kingdom

BRYAN F. MEYERS, MD, MPH
Patrick and Joy Williamson Professor of
Surgery, Department of Surgery, Washington
University School of Medicine, Saint Louis,
Missouri

DANIEL L. MILLER, MD
Kamal A. Mansour Professor of Thoracic
Surgery and Chief, General Thoracic Surgery,
Division of Cardiothoracic Surgery,
Department of Surgery, Emory University
School of Medicine, Emory University Hospital,
Atlanta, Georgia

SUDISH C. MURTHY, MD, PhD
Staff, Department of Thoracic and
Cardiovascular Surgery; and Surgical Director,
Center of Major Airway Disease, Cleveland
Clinic, Cleveland, Ohio

KEITH S. NAUNHEIM, MD
Program Director; The Valle L. and Melba
Willman Professor; and Chief, Department
of Cardiothoracic Surgery, St. Louis University
Health Sciences Center, St. Louis, Missouri

INGER OEY, MD, FRCS
Clinical Assistant, Consultant Thoracic
Surgeon, Department of Thoracic Surgery,
Glenfield Hospital, University Hospitals
of Leister–NHS Trust, Leister,
United Kingdom

G. ALEXANDER PATTERSON, MD
Evarts A. Graham Professor of Surgery and
Chief, Division of Cardiothoracic Surgery,
Washington University School of Medicine,
Barnes-Jewish Hospital, St. Louis, Missouri

MICHAEL I. POLKEY, PhD, FRCP
Professor, Department of Respiratory
Medicine, Royal Brompton Hospital, London,
United Kingdom

ERINO A. RENDINA, MD
Professor of Surgery, Université di Roma
"La Sapienza," Cattedra di Chirurgia Toracica,
Policlinico Umberto I, Rome Italy

RALPH A. SCHMID, MD
Professor of Surgery and Director, Division
of General Thoracic Surgery, University
Hospital Berne, Berne, Switzerland

PALLAV L. SHAH, MD, FRCP
Consultant Respiratory Physician, Department
of Respiratory Medicine, Royal Brompton
Hospital, London, United Kingdom

K. ROBERT SHEN, MD
Assistant Professor of Surgery, Department of
Surgery, Division of General Thoracic Surgery,
Mayo Clinic and Mayo Foundation, Rochester,
Minnesota

JOSEPH B. SHRAGER, MD
Chief, Division of Thoracic Surgery; Professor
of Cardiothoracic Surgery, Stanford University
School of Medicine, Stanford Hospitals and
Clinics, Stanford; and Veterans Affairs Palo
Alto Health Care System, Palo Alto, California

**JULIAN A. SMITH, MB, MS, FRACS,
FACS, FCSANZ**
Head, Department of Surgery (MMC), Monash
University; Head, Cardiothoracic Surgery Unit;
and Medical Director, Specialty Program,
Southern Health, Monash Medical Centre,
Clayton, Victoria, Australia

STEVEN C. SPRINGMEYER, MD
School of Medicine, University of Washington,
Seattle; and Spiration Inc., Redmond,
Washington

GERHARD W. SYBRECHT, MD
Professor of Medicine, Klinik fur Innere
Medizin, Pneumologie, Allergologie,
Beatmungs und Umweltmedizi, Meizinische
Universitatsklinik, Saarland, Germany

MICHAELA TUTIC, MD
Department of Surgery, Division of Thoracic
Surgery, University Hospital of Zurich, Zurich,
Switzerland

DIRK VAN RAEMDONCK, MD
The Lung Transplant Program, University
Hospital Gathuisberg, Leuven, Belgium

FEDERICO VENUTA, MD
Professor of Surgery, Université di Roma
"La Sapienza," Cattedra di Chirurgia Toracica,
Policlinico Umberto I, Rome Italy

THOMAS K. WADDELL, MD
Toronto Lung Transplant Program, Toronto
General Hospital, Toronto, Ontario, Canada

DAVID WALLER, MD, FRCS (CTh), FCCP
Consultant Thoracic Surgeon, Department
of Thoracic Surgery, Glenfield Hospital,
University Hospitals of Leister–NHS Trust,
Leister, United Kingdom

WALTER WEDER, MD
Professor and Chief, Department of Surgery,
Division of Thoracic Surgery, University
Hospital of Zurich, Zurich, Switzerland

DOUGLAS E. WOOD, MD
Endowed Chair of Lung Cancer Research;
Department of Thoracic Surgery, University
of Washington; and University of Washington
Medical Center, Seattle, Washington

JONATHAN C. YEUNG, MD
Toronto Lung Transplant Program, Toronto
General Hospital, Toronto, Ontario, Canada

Contents

This article presents the epidemiology, etiology, clinical features and natural history of emphysema. Emphysema is defined as abnormal, permanent enlargement of air spaces distal to the terminal bronchioles, accompanied by the destruction of their walls and without obvious fibrosis. This destruction results in the loss of acinar structure, and a subsequent reduction in the area available for gas exchange. The associated loss of elastic tissue leads to small airway collapse and the gas trapping that is often a prominent feature of the disease. The burden of disease attributable to emphysema is significant and growing, and is a leading cause of disability in middle and late life.

Emerging treatments require appropriate CT targeting of a selected lobe or lobes and target airways to obtain a successful response. CT scan is used in pretreatment planning to select patients and plan treatment strategy and posttreatment to confirm correct deployment of devices and assess treatment response. Increasingly treatments are being developed to treat patients who have emphysema who require accurate quantitation of extent and distribution of the process. Functional assessment can be made by inference of detailed anatomic correlates and by direct measurement of regional function using dynamic scan protocols. This article summarizes the current role of imaging in the assessment of patients who have emphysema.

Emphysema is a chronic and debilitating disease in which affected patients must deal with diminished quality of life and poor functional status. Because contemporary medical therapy has had little impact on mortality rates, the National Emphysema Treatment Trial was designed to provide prospective randomized evidence for the efficacy of lung volume reduction surgery. This multicenter trial showed a mortality benefit and improved function in defined subgroups of patients based on the distribution of emphysema and baseline exercise tolerance. Patients with upper-lobe predominant disease and low exercise capacity achieved the most consistent gains in survival, exercise capacity, and quality of live in the long term with lung volume reduction surgery. Other subcategories of disease distribution and baseline exercise tolerance had variable results with surgery, emphasizing the importance of patient selection in achieving good outcomes.

The current convention is for bilateral one-stage lung volume reduction surgery. Unilateral surgery results in a symptomatic improvement in most patients. A staged approach to the second lung may reduce the risk of surgery and lead to a slower decline in physiologic improvement. The timing of the second operation can be influenced by the patient and the surgeon. The surgeon may be anxious to avoid the patient becoming inoperable because of excessive physiological decline or the patient succumbing to the inherent mortal risk of emphysema. The patient may be the best arbiter. The operation should be intended to improve his or her subjective assessment of health status; therefore, this parameter ultimately should determine the surgical schedule.

performed LVRS in patients who have severe cardiac diseases. Conversely, few cardiac surgeons have been willing to undertake major cardiac surgery in patients who have severe emphysema. This report reviews the evidence regarding combined cardiac surgery and LVRS to determine the optimal management strategy for patients who have severe emphysema and who are suitable for LVRS, but who also have co-existing significant cardiac diseases that are operable.

Air leaks after pulmonary surgery represent a substantial clinical problem. When they persist beyond a few days, air leaks appear to increase complications and costs. Clearly, emphysema patients are those at greatest risk for developing problematic air leaks. This article, after reviewing what is known about the epidemiology and clinical significance of air leaks, discusses the various techniques that may be employed to avoid the development of problematic air leaks and to manage them when they do occur. It reviews the data available on newer and more traditional options for the prophylaxis and management of air leaks and offers the authors' opinions about the optimal approaches in various clinical situations.

In patients who have advanced emphysema, development of a spontaneous pneumothorax can be a life-threatening event, warranting more aggressive management. Patients who have the most advanced stages of emphysema are at the highest risk to develop spontaneous pneumothoraces, have recurrences, and are the most difficult patients to treat. Early surgical intervention should be recommended for patients who have persistent or large air leaks or those who lack parietal-to-visceral pleural apposition after a trial of nonoperative management. Video-assisted thoracoscopy with resection of the offending bulla and pleurodesis or pleurectomy also should be considered to prevent recurrences in all patients with chronic obstructive pulmonary disease who are safe operative candidates.

Airway bypass is a new form of minimally invasive therapy for the treatment of homogeneous emphysema. It is a bronchoscopic catheter-based therapy that forms transbronchial extra-anatomic passages at the bronchial segmental or subsegmental level. The passages are expanded and supported and the patency is maintained by paclitaxel drug-eluting airway bypass stents. This article provides an overview of airway bypass, outlining its concept, development, and experimental studies, and briefly describes the current multicenter, prospective, randomized, double-blind trial evaluating airway bypass, the Exhale Airway Stents for Emphysema (EASE) Trial.

Ninety-eight emphysema patients were treated at 13 international sites during a 3-year series of single-arm, open-label studies with the IBV valve and a multi-lobar treatment approach. Fifty six percent of subjects had a clinically meaningful improvement in health-related quality of life, but standard pulmonary function and exercise studies were insensitive effectiveness measures. Quantitative CT analyses of regional lung changes showed lobar volume changes in over 85% of subjects. Lung volume reduction was an uncommon mechanism for a treatment response with bilateral upper lobe treatment. A redirection of inspired air, an interlobar shift to healthier lung tissue, was the most common mechanism for a valve treatment response.

Numerous endoscopic procedures have recently been studied and progressively introduced in clinical practice to improve mechanics and function in patients who have emphysema. Bronchoscopic lung volume reduction with one-way endobronchial valves facilitates deflation of the most overinflated emphysematous parts of the lung. These valves have been designed to control and redirect airflow by preventing air from entering the target parenchymal area but allowing air and mucus to exit. The preliminary results have shown that this procedure is safe and effective at medium term in a selected group of patients.

The shortage of adequate organ donors remains a major challenge in clinical lung transplantation. Use of lungs from non–heart-beating donors has been used to increase the number of lung donors. By expanding the criteria for donor lung selection and by using novel approaches for lung assessment, it is anticipated that the rate of lung utilization will also improve. Ultimately, it is hoped that the repair of injured donor lungs ex vivo will further increase the rate of lung utilization to the point of meeting the demand.

Significant improvements in human lung transplantation have occurred since the first successful single lung transplant in 1983 and the first bilateral transplant in 1986. Despite improvements with donor selection, challenges remain in lung preservation, recipient prioritization, perioperative mortality, and long-term morbidity. In an effort to optimize the benefits derived from lung transplantation, the United Network for Organ Sharing (UNOS) recently reorganized the prioritization scheme by which potential recipients were listed. The focus of this article is to review the current status of lung transplantation for emphysema, with attention given to current outcomes and management strategies.

Thoracic Surgery Clinics

THE CLINICS ARE NOW AVAILABLE ONLINE!

Access your subscription at:
www.theclinics.com

Preface

Progress in the Surgical and Endoscopic Treatment of Emphysema: Where Are We Now?

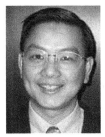

Cliff K. Choong, MBBS, FRACS, FRCS
Guest Editor

Severe emphysema is a debilitating condition and, in a majority of the patients, is secondary to the effects of smoking. Patho-physiologically, there is destruction of alveolar walls, permanent enlargement of alveoli and alveolar ducts, damage to parenchymal tissues, reduced mechanical support of airways, and expiratory flow collapse. This leads to extensive gas trapping, severe hyperinflation, and a marked impairment of chest wall and diaphragmatic movements, resulting in impaired gas exchange and difficulty breathing. Clinically, patients present with increasing dyspnea after mild exertion or even at rest, and they become progressively restricted in the ability to carry out normal living activities. Significant mortality is also seen in patients with a mean forced expiratory volume in 1 second (FEV_1) of 1L (mortality 10% per year) and $FEV_1 < 0.75$L (5 year survival is 25%).[1] Emphysema is a common problem and affects approximately 2 million individuals in the United States and is the fourth leading cause of death.[2] The World Health Organization (WHO) estimates that 210 million people worldwide suffer from the disease, and that it led to over 3 million deaths globally in 2005 (5% of all deaths).[3] Current medical treatment is generally limited to palliative measures that include smoking cessation, supplemental oxygen, bronchodilators, anti-inflammatory drugs, and pulmonary rehabilitation.

Five decades ago, in 1959, Brantigan and colleagues[4] suggested that partial pulmonary resection could produce symptomatic and functional improvement in some patients who had emphysema. Brantigan did his operation through a standard thoracotomy, performing multiple lung resections and plications, and incorporating radical hilar stripping to denervate the lung. This latter component, it was thought, reduced the production of tenacious sputum.[4] This procedure resulted in high mortality and modest clinical benefit and did not gain wide acceptance. In 1995, Cooper and colleagues[5] undertook bilateral lung volume reduction surgery (LVRS) in 20 patients who had severe chronic obstructive pulmonary disease (COPD) to relieve thoracic distension and improve respiratory mechanics. The operation was performed through a median sternotomy and involved excision of 20% to 30% of the volume of each lung. The most affected portions were excised with the use of a linear stapling device buttressed with bovine pericardial strips to eliminate air leakage through the staple holes. There was no early or late mortality and no requirement for immediate postoperative ventilatory assistance. At a mean follow-up of 6.4 months, the patients experienced an improvement in mean FEV_1 of 82%. There were also significant improvements in total lung capacity, residual volume (RV), and trapped gas. The changes were

Thorac Surg Clin 19 (2009) xiii–xvi
doi:10.1016/j.thorsurg.2009.04.005

associated with marked relief of dyspnea and improvement in exercise tolerance and quality of life.[5] Although the follow-up period was short, these preliminary results suggested that bilateral LVRS may be of significant value for selected patients who have severe COPD. In 2003, the same group reported the long-term survival and functional results of 250 consecutive patients after bilateral LVRS.[6] The in-hospital mortality was 4.8%, and the median length of hospitalization was 9 days. At a median follow-up of 4.4 years, the patients had significant improvements in FEV_1 and RV between preoperative values and each time point of follow-up. Health-related quality of life showed significant postoperative improvement and, with time, correlated well with the improvement in FEV_1. The Kaplan-Meier survivals after LVRS for the group of patients were 93.6%, 84.4%, and 67.7% at 1, 3, and 5 years, respectively. The study therefore found that LVRS produces significant functional improvement for selected patients who have emphysema and, for most of these patients, the benefits appear to last at least 5 years.[6]

The National Emphysema Treatment Trial (NETT) is a prospective randomized study that evaluated outcomes of patients randomized to either medical therapy or bilateral LVRS.[7–10] The design and rationale was finalized in 1997/1998; screening and enrollment began in October of 1997 and randomization began in January of 1998.[7] Of the 3777 patients screened for the NETT, 2559 were ineligible and 1218 patients were randomized.[7,8] The NETT identified and published, in 2001, a subgroup of patients who had low FEV_1 <20% plus homogenous emphysema or low DLCO <20% to be at increased risk of mortality following LVRS (16%) over medical therapy (0%).[9] There was also limited functional improvement in this subgroup of patients following LVRS. The initial full report of the NETT was published in 2003 and demonstrated a significant survival benefit from LVRS in patients with upper lobe-predominant emphysema and low exercise capacity.[8] The upper lobe-predominant patients treated with LVRS also demonstrated significant benefits in exercise improvement and dyspnea compared with their medically treated counterparts, and the non–upper lobe-predominant LVRS treated patients with low exercise capacity had improvement in dyspnea. Other subgroups were noted to be "high risk," with high mortality after surgery and were not offset by improvements in exercise capacity or quality of life, and therefore were considered to be poor LVRS candidates.[8,9] These reports were made on the basis of a median follow up of 2.4 years. Report on the long term

follow up of these patients was published in 2006 and provided an updated analysis of 4.3 years median follow up and included 40% more patients with functional measures 2 years after randomization.[10] There was an overall survival advantage for LVRS, with a 5-year risk ratio (RR) for death of 0.86. Improvement was more likely in the LVRS than in the medical group for maximal exercise through 3 years and for health-related quality of life (St. George's Respiratory Questionnaire [SGRQ]) through 4 years. Updated comparisons of survival and functional improvement were consistent with initial results for four clinical subgroups of non–high-risk patients defined by upper lobe predominance and exercise capacity.[9,10] After LVRS, the upper-lobe patients with low exercise capacity demonstrated improved survival (5-year RR, 0.67), exercise throughout 3 years, and symptoms (SGRQ) through 5 years. The upper-lobe-predominant and high-exercise-capacity LVRS patients did not obtain any survival advantage but were likely to improve their exercise capacity and SGRQ. The study therefore found that the effects of LVRS are durable, and it can be recommended for upper lobe-predominant emphysema patients with low exercise capacity and should be considered for palliation in patients with upper lobe emphysema and high exercise capacity.[9,10] In this issue of *Thoracic Surgery Clinics*, a summary of the NETT is provided together with other aspects of LVRS: staged LVRS, LVRS for nonheterogenous emphysema, and LVRS for alpha-1 antitrypsin deficiency emphysema. Intraoperative and postoperative management of air leaks in patients who have emphysema, and decision making in the management of secondary spontaneous pneumothorax in patients who have severe emphysema are clinically relevant in the management of emphysematous patients and are also covered in this issue.

Endoscopic management of emphysema is a new form of minimally invasive therapy that is undergoing clinical evaluation. Some have termed it as bronchoscopic lung volume reduction (BLVR). There are two different concepts. The first concept is the utilization of one way endobronchial valves that are placed within the lumen of airways allowing air to flow only unidirectionally out of the airways (ie, air flow in the direction of expiration) and does not allow air to be inspired through the valves. The endobronchial valves are available in variable sizes to allow placement within different airway luminal sizes. The aim is to completely collapse a hyperinflated lobe of the lung by placing several endobronchial valves to occlude all the segmental or subsegmental airways supplying the specific lobe. This form of therapy is targeted at patients who have heterogenous emphysema. The valves are placed bronchoscopically through the working channel of a flexible bronchoscope and they are removable. There are two different companies that produce these one-way endobronchial valves. Though the valve designs are different between the two companies, they both share some common features, as described above. The companies are Emphasys Medical Inc. (Redwood City, California), which produces the Emphasys Zephyr Endobronchial Valve (EBV), and Spiration Inc. (Redmond, Washington), which produces the the IBV Valve.[11,12]

The second concept is airway bypass. Airway bypass is the creation of noncollapsing, extra-anatomic passages that connect lung parenchyma to large airways.[13–19] It takes advantage of the increased collateral ventilation in emphysematous patients to bypass collapsing and obstructed small airways, thereby allowing trapped gas to escape and reduce hyperinflation. Collateral ventilation is the ability of gas to move from one part of the lung to another through nonanatomic pathways. This has been demonstrated to be greatly increased in emphysema, because of the extensive breakdown of alveolar walls and lobular septae. Airway bypass is a minimally invasive treatment with the potential to improve pulmonary function and reduce dyspnea in patients who have homogeneous emphysema.[13–19] This concept is in contrast to the endobronchial valves, which are targeting patients who have heterogenous emphysema. In airway bypass, transbronchial passages are created between segmental or subsegmental bronchi and adjacent lung parenchyma, and these are reinforced with a paclitaxel-eluting airway bypass stent. The purpose of the drug component of the stent is to prevent occlusion of the stented transbronchial passages. The airway bypass stent is manufactured by Broncus Technologies Inc. (Mountain View, California), which produces the "Exhale Emphysema Treatment System."[19] Clinical trials of the various endobronchial devices and the airway bypass stents are presently ongoing. This issue of *Thoracic Surgery Clinics* provides a review on the different endoscopic treatment modalities for emphysema.

Lung transplantation is a useful therapeutic option for highly selected patients who have end-stage lung failure. Patients with successful transplantation experience an improvement in pulmonary function indices, exercise performance, and quality of life. This issue of *Thoracic Surgery Clinics* provides an update on lung transplantation for emphysema and an update on donor assessment, resuscitation, and acceptance criteria, including novel techniques such as non–heart beating donor lung retrieval and ex vivo donor lung perfusion.

This issue of *Thoracic Surgery Clinics* provides a comprehensive review and update on the surgical and endoscopic management of emphysema. The aspects covered include the epidemiology and pathophysiology of emphysema, an update on radiology imaging of emphysema and therapeutic implications, the various aspects of LVRS, endoscopic management of emphysema, and an update on donor lung retrieval and lung transplantation for emphysema.

Cliff K. Choong, MBBS, FRACS, FRCS
Department of Surgery
Monash University
Block E, Level 5
Monash Medical Centre
246 Clayton Road
Clayton, Victoria 3168
Australia

E-mail address:
cliffchoong@hotmail.com

REFERENCES

1. Deiner CV, Burrows B. Further observations on the course and prognosis of chronic obstructive lung disease. Am Rev Respir Dis 1975;3:719.
2. Snider G, Kleinerman J, Thurlbeck W, et al. The definition of emphysema. Report of a National Heart, Lung, and Blood Institute, Division of Lung Disease Workshop. Am Rev Respir Dis 1985;132:182–5.
3. World Health Organization. Chronic obstructive pulmonary disease. Fact sheet No. 315. Geneva (Switzerland): World Health Organization; 2008.
4. Brantigan OC, Mueller E, Kress MB. A surgical approach to pulmonary emphysema. Am Rev Respir Dis 1959;80:194–202.
5. Cooper JD, Trulock EP, Triantafillou AN, et al. Bilateral pneumonectomy (volume reduction) for chronic obstructive pulmonary disease. J Thorac Cardiovasc Surg 1995;109:106–19.
6. Ciccone AM, Meyers BF, Guthrie TJ, et al. Long-term outcome of bilateral lung volume reduction in 250 consecutive patients with emphysema. J Thorac Cardiovasc Surg 2003;125(3):513–25.
7. National Emphysema Treatment Trial Research Group Rationale and design of the National Emphysema Treatment Trial (NETT): a prospective randomized trial of lung volume reduction surgery. J Thorac Cardiovasc Surg 1999;118:518–28.
8. Fishman A, Martinez F, Naunheim K, et al. A randomized trial comparing LVRS with medical therapy for

severe emphysema. N Engl J Med 2003;348: 2059–73.

9. Fishman A, Fessler H, Martinez F, et al. Patients at high risk of death after lung-volume reduction surgery. N Engl J Med 2001;345(15):1075–83.

10. Naunheim KS, Wood DE, Mohsenifar Z, et al. the National Emphysema Treatment Trial Research Group. Long-term follow-up of patients receiving lung-volume-reduction surgery versus medical therapy for severe emphysema by the National Emphysema Treatment Trial Research Group. Ann Thorac Surg 2006;82:431–43.

11. Emphasys Medical Inc., Redwood City, California. Available at: http://www.emphasysmedical.com/index.cfm. Accessed January 1, 2009.

12. Spiration Inc., Redmond, WA. Available at: http://www.spirationinc.com/index.asp. Accessed January 1, 2009.

13. Lausberg HF, Chino K, Patterson GA, et al. Bronchial fenestration improves expiratory flow in emphysematous human lungs. Ann Thorac Surg 2003;75:393–7.

14. Choong CK, Macklem PT, Pierce JA, et al. Airway bypass improves the mechanical properties of explanted emphysematous lungs. Am J Respir Crit Care Med 2008;178:902–5.

15. Choong CK, Haddad FJ, Gee EY, et al. Feasibility and safety of airway bypass stent placement and influence of topical mitomycin C on stent patency. J Thorac Cardiovasc Surg 2005;129:632–8.

16. Choong CK, Phan L, Massetti P, et al. Prolongation of patency of airway bypass stents with use of drug-eluting stents. J Thorac Cardiovasc Surg 2006;131:60–4.

17. Rendina EA, De Giacomo T, Venuta F, et al. Feasibility and safety of the airway bypass procedure for patients with emphysema. J Thorac Cardiovasc Surg 2003;125:1294–9.

18. Cardoso PFG, Snell GI, Hopkins P, et al. Clinical application of airway bypass with paclitaxel-eluting stents: early results. J Thorac Cardiovasc Surg 2007;134:974–81.

19. Broncus Technologies Inc., Mountain View, California. Available at: http://www.broncus.com/default.asp. Accessed January 1, 2009.

The Epidemiology, Etiology, Clinical Features, and Natural History of Emphysema

Samuel V. Kemp, MBBS, MRCP*, Michael I. Polkey, PhD, FRCP,
Pallav L. Shah, MD, FRCP

KEYWORDS
- Emphysema • Chronic obstructive pulmonary disease
- Smoking • Etiology • Natural history

DEFINITION AND HISTORY OF EMPHYSEMA

The term emphysema derives directly from the Greek word emphysēma, meaning inflation (from the verb emphysaein, to inflate, or blow in). It is defined as abnormal, permanent enlargement of air spaces distal to the terminal bronchioles, accompanied by the destruction of their walls and without obvious fibrosis. This destruction results in the loss of acinar structure, and a subsequent reduction in the area available for gas exchange (**Fig. 1**). The associated loss of elastic tissue leads to small airway collapse and the gas trapping that is often a prominent feature of the disease. Clinically, emphysema is part of the spectrum of disease encompassed by the term "chronic obstructive pulmonary disease" (COPD) that also covers chronic bronchitis, which is a chronic productive cough for 3 months during each of 2 consecutive years (other causes of cough being excluded). The cardinal feature of both emphysema and bronchitis is airflow obstruction.

Frederick Ruysch,[1] a professor of botany in Amsterdam and famous for his human anatomic preparations, as well as discovering many anatomic structures (including the bronchial vessels) provided the first recognized description of emphysema in 1691 (**Fig. 2**). In the 1799 engravings published to illustrate his famous work, *The Morbid Anatomy of Some of the Most Important Parts of the Human Body*, Matthew Baillie[2,3] produced the first detailed illustrations of

emphysema. Subsequent work by great minds such as Laennec[4] and Orsos[5] further characterized the disease, with the realization that disruption of the elastic fibers of the distal airways was the primary underlying pathology.

The recognition of different pathologically patterns of emphysema first came about from the work of Gough and colleagues[6,7] in Cardiff in the 1950s, and can now be divided into three subtypes: centrilobular, panacinar, and paraseptal. Centrilobular emphysema is characterized by the loss of respiratory bronchioles with a degree of sparing of the distal alveoli, and predominantly affects the upper portions of the lung. This pattern is the one that is most commonly seen in smokers. Panacinar emphysema affects the entire acinus uniformly; is seen predominantly in the lower lobes; and is the pattern most associated with α-1 antitrypsin deficiency. Paraseptal (also known as distal acinar) emphysema is localized around the septae and pluera, and affects the distal acinar structures. Although often co-existing with centrilobular emphysema in smokers, it can be an incidental finding in young patients and may lead to spontaneous pneumothorax, particularly in apical disease. Bullous emphysema develops from the local expansion of air spaces owing to air trapping, and, in giant bullous disease, can cause significant compression of remaining lung tissue.

However, the distribution on imaging rather than the histologic pattern of disease is probably more useful clinically, because lung volume reduction

Department of Respiratory Medicine, Royal Brompton Hospital, Sydney Street, London SW3 6NP, UK
* Corresponding author.
E-mail address: s.kemp@rbhnt.nhs.uk (S.V. Kemp).

Thorac Surg Clin 19 (2009) 149–158
doi:10.1016/j.thorsurg.2009.03.003

thoracic.theclinics.com

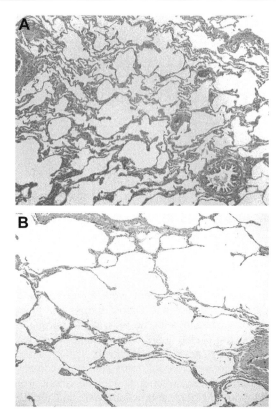

Fig. 1. Panel *A* shows normal lung tissue. Panel *B* demonstrates the loss of alveolar structures and of surface area in emphysema (both x40). (*Courtesy of* Augustine G. DiGiovanna, Salisbury University, Salisbury, MD; with permission. Copyright © 2004. All rights reserved.)

surgery has been shown to benefit those with a predominance of upper lobe disease,[8] and endobronchial valve trials have been designed with this same patient group in mind.[9,10]

DIAGNOSIS

The Global Initiative for Chronic Obstructive Lung Disease (GOLD) defines COPD as "a preventable and treatable disease with some significant extrapulmonary effects that may contribute to the severity in individual patients. Its pulmonary component is characterized by airflow limitation that is not fully reversible. The airflow limitation is usually progressive and associated with an abnormal inflammatory response of the lung to noxious particles or gases." This definition recognizes the permanent loss of lung function, as well as the often-neglected nonpulmonary components of the disease. The diagnosis of COPD relies on spirometric measurements of forced vital capacity (FVC) and post-bronchodilator forced expiratory volume in 1 second (FEV_1), the most

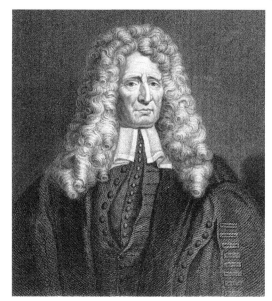

Fig. 2. Picture of Ruysch (credited with the first written description of emphysema).

widely used criteria being those defined by GOLD. The diagnosis requires an FEV_1/FVC ratio of <0.7, and patients are then stratified into four categories from mild to very severe disease based on the severity of FEV_1 impairment as set out in **Table 1** below.[11] The original GOLD publication separated moderate disease into stage IIa and IIb,[12] but the staging was later changed such that IIb has become III (severe) and stage IV (very severe) has been added. More recently, the National Institute for Health and Clinical Excellence (NICE) in the United Kingdom has published its own guidelines, which differ slightly from the GOLD criteria.[13] While maintaining the need for an FEV_1/FVC ratio of <0.7, it has done away with the most mild category of disease all together, with an FEV_1 of <80% predicted required to establish the diagnosis.

As the degree of airflow obstruction increases, so too, in general, does the degree of physical limitation and frequency of exacerbations, although there is considerable individual variation in symptom severity.

EPIDEMIOLOGY

COPD is a common and under-diagnosed problem. The World Health Organization (WHO) estimates that 210 million people worldwide suffer from the disease, and that it led to over 3 million deaths globally in 2005 (5% of all deaths).[14] It is thought that around half of all COPD cases in the developed world remain undiagnosed, and this proportion is likely to be higher still in the

Table 1
Chronic obstructive pulmonary disease staging by FEV$_1$

GOLD Staging		NICE Staging	
Stage I: Mild	FEV$_1$/FVC <70% FEV$_1$ ≥80% predicted	Airflow limitation not meeting criteria for a diagnosis of COPD	
Stage II: Moderate	FEV$_1$/FVC <70% FEV$_1$ <80% predicted	Mild	FEV$_1$/FVC <70% FEV$_1$ <80% predicted
Stage III: Severe	FEV$_1$/FVC <70% FEV$_1$ <50% predicted	Moderate	FEV$_1$/FVC <70% FEV$_1$ <50% predicted
Stage IV: Very severe	FEV$_1$/FVC <70% FEV$_1$ <30% predicted or FEV$_1$ <50% predicted with chronic respiratory failure	Severe	FEV$_1$/FVC <70% FEV$_1$ <30% predicted

developing world. Data from NHANES III[15] indicated that, at the end of the 20th century, 24 million Americans were living with impaired lung function, with 10 million of those reporting physician-diagnosed COPD. Eight million physician consultations, 1.5 million emergency department attendances, and 726,000 hospital admissions were attributed to COPD, with 119,000 deaths. Similar data is available for England and Wales, and the most robust recent data estimates 900,000 people with a diagnosis COPD,[16] although the true number is likely to be closer to 2 million. Over 100,000 admissions account for over 1 million bed-days, and the disease is thought to cost the National Health Service nearly £1.5 billion annually,[13] a huge strain on the public purse.

The accumulation of tobacco smoking (or other risk factor exposure) required to cause destructive lung disease means that emphysema is predominantly a disease of middle and late adult life. Disease is often seen earlier in α1-antitrypsin deficiency, especially in those who also smoke, but isolated cases of early onset smoking-related disease in the absence of α1-antitrypsin deficiency are occasionally seen.[17]

Historically, COPD has been a male-dominated disease, but the increase in female smokers in the developed world and the increased risk of exposure to biomass fuels in developing countries has led to an equal distribution between the sexes. 90% of all deaths from COPD are thought to occur in the developing world,[14] where health care systems are absent or insufficient. This situation is mirrored to some extent in developed countries, were there is an association with lower social class. Many factors play a role here, and include smoking status, occupational history (manual labor and exposure to dusts and fumes), and poorer utilization of available health resources.

ETIOLOGY
Tobacco Smoke

Tobacco smoking is by far the single most important factor in the development of emphysema, and accounts for 80%–90% of cases in the developed world. The decline in FEV$_1$ with smoking was shown by Fletcher and Peto in 1977,[18] but they had suggested that only a minority of smokers would go on to develop clinically significant airflow obstruction. This analysis led to the erroneous belief that there were effectively two populations of smokers: those who were resistant and those who were susceptible. Subsequent work over the years has shown that the amount of tobacco smoked is strongly correlated to the degree of emphysema and airflow obstruction, and it is now increasingly apparent that there is a continuum of susceptibility which is likely due to the interplay of a number of genetic and other environmental factors.

The increasing use of cannabis has led to the recognition of emphysematous lung disease, often bullous in nature, in some users. The degree to which lung destruction can be attributed to the cannabis itself is uncertain, however, as studies are confounded by the mixing of the drug with tobacco when smoking, and the use of deeper inhalation and breath holding for maximal effect.

Genetics

The most well-known genetic association with emphysema is that of α-1 antitrypsin deficiency, discovered in 1963 by Carl-Bertil Laurell,[19] a remarkable biochemist known for his discoveries of transferring,[20] caeruloplasmin,[21] and haptoglobin,[22] and for a crucial role in the description of Waldenström's macroglobulinaemia (named after his collaborator).[23] In addition to its importance in the field of emphysema, the discovery led to the identification of a new class of conformational protease inhibitors, the serpins, crucial in many biologic processes including coagulation and inflammation. A detailed discussion of the condition is beyond the scope of this article, but a brief description of the more important aspects follows.

The α1-antitrypsin gene is found on chromosome 14, and α1-antitrypsin is produced in the liver. Mutations of this gene lead to abnormal protein folding with altered secretion from hepatocytes, and subsequent low circulating blood levels. α1-antitrypsin is a wide-ranging antiprotease, but its most relevant activity in respect to the lungs is its action against neutrophil elastase, released from neutrophils at areas of inflammation and in response to tobacco smoke. A lack of α1-antitrypsin allows unopposed elastase activity and subsequent destruction of the lung architecture. While previously thought to be largely a disease affecting those of European descent, it is now recognized that the disease affects a wide range of geographic and ethnic populations.[24]

There are over 75 alleles of the α1-antitrypsin gene (designated Pi).[25] The normal allele is PiM, with PiS and PiZ the two most common abnormal expressions. It appears that only one normal allele is required to produce a normalphenotype, even though these individuals (PiMS, PiMZ) have lower serum α1-antitrypsin levels than PiMM individuals. Apart from very rare null alleles, PiZZ is associated with the most severe clinical picture, as not only are levels severely reduced, but the activity of the gene product is also diminished. The onset of clinical disease is variable, but it is usually evident by the fifth or sixth decade, and roughly 20 years earlier in those who smoke.[26]

Many other genes have been implicated in the pathogenesis of emphysema. Hersh and colleagues[27] have identified single nucleotide polymorphisms associated with different clinical features of advanced emphysema, including dyspnoea (transforming growth factor-beta1 [TGFB1]), exercise tolerance (latent transforming growth factor-beta binding protein-4 [LTBP4]), and gas transfer impairment (epoxyhydrolase 1 [EPHX1]), and gene polymorphisms in glutathione S-transferase p1 (GSTP1), EPHX1, and matrix metalloproteinase 1 (MMP1) have recently been shown to be correlate with upper-lobe predominant disease. This last finding is interesting, as altered function in these xenobiotic enzymes may alter detoxification of cigarette smoke metabolites.[28]

Early-Life Influences

Although emphysema is traditionally thought of as an adult disease, there is mounting evidence that early-life events are important in the development of disease in later life. Prenatal exposure to cigarette smoking is associated with measurable and significant declines in mid-expiratory flow rates (and to a lesser degree FEV_1) in childhood,[29] but whether this leads to increased susceptibility to the effects of subsequent smoking is not known. There has also been interest in the role of childhood respiratory infections in the etiology of emphysema. In 1994 the MRC Environmental Epidemiology Unit published compelling data showing the relationship between childhood pneumonia and impaired FEV_1 in adulthood,[30] although recently published data from the British 1958 Birth Cohort, suggest that the rate of decline in lung function in midadult life is unaffected.[31]

Bronchopulmonary dysplasia, a disease of prematurity in neonates treated with oxygen and mechanical ventilation, leads to airflow obstruction, hyperinflation, and areas of emphysema on CT in those who survive to adulthood.[32] Although rare, it is likely to become an increasingly frequent cause of obstructive lung disease in the adult respiratory clinic.

Industry

It has become clear that a higher prevalence of emphysema is seen in workers in several occupations associated with exposure to fumes, chemicals, and dusts. The most extensively researched of these is the coal industry, with reports as far back as the late 1940s.[33,34] Exposure to respirable dust particles ($P<.001$) and α-quartz ($P = .02$) in Norwegian tunnel workers was shown to result in an excess decline in FEV_1 of 25-38ml/yr in nonsmoking workers,[35] and studies in gold miners have demonstrated higher rates of emphysema at post-mortem in those with long term exposure to underground mineral dust.[36,37] Many such examples exist in the literature, and it is likely that any occupation in which workers are chronically exposed to a mixture of noxious fumes and airborne particles will confer an additional risk of emphysema on those workers, and this effect seems particularly prominent in those who also smoke. Knowledge of such associations is important when giving advice about continued employment, and often compensation issues arise.

Biomass Fuels

Indoor exposure to smoke from biomass fuels (wood, crop residues, charcoal, and dung) used for cooking and heating is now recognized as a major cause of COPD worldwide, and causes widespread emphysema on CT imaging.[38] It kills 1.6 million people every year of whom one million are children, and the WHO estimates that it is responsible for 22% of all cases of COPD.[39] The problem is disproportionately prevalent in women in the developing world, who can spend many hours a day around the cooking fire. A survey of over 20,000 citizens in southern China found an excess of COPD in those with poor ventilation in the kitchen and previous exposure to biomass fuels, with a degree of risk similar to a 15–30 pack year smoking history.[40]

British versus Dutch Hypothesis

The Dutch hypothesis, as it became known, postulated that asthma and COPD existed as part of a spectrum of lung disease ("chronic nonspecific lung disease") that resulted from any number of airway irritants leading to inflammation and declines in lung function. This theory seems appealing when one considers those patients with COPD with a degree of reversibility, or those with progressive asthma symptoms; however, inflammatory mediators in the two conditions are very different. An alternative theory, the British hypothesis, suggested that chronic airflow obstruction in smokers was a result of recurrent airway infections, with those getting more frequent infective episodes having the more rapid decline in lung function. This theory was discounted some 17 years later after a study by Fletcher and colleagues,[41] but it has recently been revived with reports of more rapid lung function decline in those with recurrent respiratory tract infection[42] and higher sputum bacterial counts.[43]

PATHOPHYSIOLOGY AND CLINICAL FEATURES

The inhalation of noxious particles and fumes leads to a disruption of the mucociliary escalator, inflammation, and tissue damage resulting in airflow obstruction and a variable degree of chronic sputum production. Lung defenses are altered, and there is a greater susceptibility to bacterial infection and colonization, exacerbations and perpetuation of the inflammatory process, and impaired quality of life.

On pulmonary function testing, there are reductions in all dynamic lung volumes, and graphical representations of flow and volume are characteristic. There is a scalloping of the expiratory flow-volume loop, with an increasingly severe and early pressure-dependent small airway collapse and flow reduction as the disease progresses. In contrast, static lung volumes show hyperinflation with increases in total lung capacity (TLC) and residual volume (RV), and gas trapping is manifested as an elevated RV/TLC ratio. These features lead to the typical chest radiograph of large lung volumes, hyperlucent lung fields, and flattened diaphragms (**Fig. 3**). The elastic recoil forces of the lung and the outward elastic forces of the chest wall are in equilibrium at functional residual capacity (FRC). With the slowly progressive destruction of lung tissue that underlies emphysema, the recoil forces of the lung become diminished, and FRC is shifted along the lungs compliance curve of the lungs to the detriment of pulmonary mechanics. This situation is exacerbated during exercise when ventilatory requirements are increased. Airflow obstruction and prolonged expiratory time mean that expiration cannot be completed before the urge to inspire, with inhalation triggered before FRC is reached. This dynamic leads to "stacking" of breaths and a gradual hyperinflation of the lungs, known as dynamic hyperinflation. Work of breathing is subsequently increased via two mechanisms. Firstly, the rightwards shift along the compliance curve requires a larger change in pressure (and hence effort) to generate a comparable tidal volume (V_T). Secondly, the creation of an artificially high end-expiratory lung volume, or dynamic FRC, means that residual elastic recoil forces must be overcome before negative intrathoracic pressures are generated and inspiratory airflow can begin: intrinsic PEEP (PEEPi). These mechanisms are illustrated in **Fig. 4**.

The loss of distal airway structures reduces the effective surface area of the lung and hence the area available for gas exchange, and the associated disruption of the alveolar-capillary architecture over

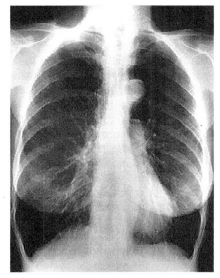

Fig. 3. Typical chest radiograph of a patient with emphysema demonstrating the hyperexpansion, hypertransradiance, and flattened diaphragms caused by air trapping.

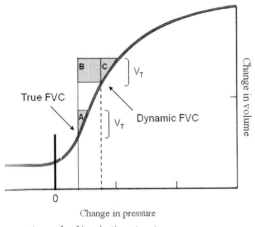

A: work of inspiration at rest
B: work of overcoming PEEPi
C: work of inspiration at dynamic FRC

Fig. 4. Compliance curve of the lung.

time leads to ventilation-perfusion (V/Q) mismatch. As arterial carbon dioxide (CO_2) levels are inversely correlated with alveolar ventilation, CO_2 levels can initially be maintained in the face of hypoxia by an increase in the minute volume. As the disease advances, there is an increase in physiologic dead-space secondary to under-perfused alveoli, and the subsequent impairment of CO_2 clearance results in hypercapnic respiratory failure.

Pulmonary arterial hypertension (PAH) may develop in any severe lung disease, and thus is seen in patients with advanced emphysema, exacerbating breathlessness and worsening exercise tolerance. There appears to be a subgroup of patients in whom there is a disproportionate degree of PAH,[44] the mechanisms for which are not clear but may be genetic in origin.[45] Although there has been burgeoning interest in the use of pulmonary vasodilators in patients with secondary PAH, robust evidence for their use is lacking. Nonetheless, a referral to an expert in the field should be considered for those with significant or symptomatic PAH for enrollment in clinical trials.

Increasing recognition has been given to the nonpulmonary aspects of obstructive airways disease over recent years. Arguably the most important of these is peripheral muscle weakness, particularly of the quadriceps muscles, the strength of which has been shown to predict mortality in moderate to severe COPD.[46] The etiology appears to be multifactorial, including disuse atrophy, the effects of systemic steroid therapy, and genetic factors. Work by Hopkinson and colleagues[47] has shown associations between quadriceps strength and genotypes of the angiotensin converting enzyme (ACE) and

vitamin D receptors,[48] potentially exciting targets for future therapies.

Collateral ventilation is the ventilation of alveolar structures through passages or channels that bypass the normal airways, and occurs through interalveolar (pores of Kohn, who originally thought them pathological[49]), bronchioloalveolar (channels of Lambert), and interbronchiolar (channels of Martin) connections. These high-resistance channels are clinically unimportant in health, but as airflow obstruction increases in the emphysematous lung, airways resistance approaches collateral resistance and collateral airflow increases.[50] This recruitment of collateral channels is assisted by hyperinflation, because there is an inverse relationship between resistance in collateral channels and lung volume.[51] With the advent of endobronchial valve treatments for upper-lobe predominant heterogeneous emphysema, there is a renewed interest in measurements of collateral ventilation. Results from the endobronchial *V*alves for *E*mphysema palliatio*N* *T*rial (VENT; Sciurba F, unpublished data, 2007) showed that those with incomplete fissures on lung CT did not derive the same degree of benefit from valve placement as those with complete fissures, the inference being that collateral channels continued to aerate the treated segments preventing volume loss.

NATURAL HISTORY

COPD is recognized as a progressive disease, both in terms of symptoms and clinical measures of disease activity. Those with GOLD stage I disease usually have no symptoms or signs, in keeping with the very mild degree of airflow limitation. Symptoms then largely progress as outlined below, although there is considerable individual variation.

Stage II
> No abnormal signs, have little or no breathlessness, and symptoms are limited to a "smoker's cough."

Stage III
> Onset of breathlessness with or without wheeze on moderate exertion, a productive cough, and abnormal signs such as a general reduction in breath sounds and the presence of wheeze.

Stage IV
> Breathlessness on any exertion and even at rest, with prominent wheeze and cough, hyperinflation, and the eventual development of cyanosis, peripheral edema and polycythaemia, especially during exacerbations.

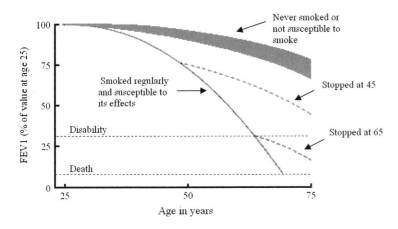

Fig. 5. Decline in FEV1 with age and smoking. (*Adapted from* Fletcher C, Peto R. The natural history of chronic airflow obstruction. Br Med J 1977;1:1645–8; with permission from BMJ Publishing Group.)

Never-smokers show a loss of FEV_1 at approximately 40 mls per year but almost never reach a level at which they are disabled by reduced airflow. Even in light smokers, there is an additional accelerated decline, and a similar relationship almost certainly exists with exposure to any number of noxious stimuli, but a return to the usual age-related decline is seen on their withdrawal.[18] There may also be an accelerated loss with advancing age.[52] As lung function is already impaired on removal of any exposure, the subsequent natural fall results in development of worsening disability, as illustrated in **Fig. 5**.

As emphysema comes under the umbrella of COPD, there is limited information on the natural history of emphysema per se. The National Emphysema Treatment Trial (NETT)[8] resulted in the collection of a large amount of follow-up data on this specific population of patients, with information regarding progression of lung function, symptoms, health status, exercise capacity, and mortality. The May 2008 issue of the Proceedings of the American Thoracic Society published a series of articles analyzing this data, and the findings are summarized below.

COPD patients are known to have an impaired quality of life, which worsens with deterioration of lung function[53] and time,[54] findings that were replicated in the NETT.[55] Those patients treated medically also had a progressive decline in exercise capacity as measured by cycle ergometry. Mortality was correlated with a number of clinical and physiologic measures. Higher RV and lower TLC were independently predictive of mortality in multivariate analysis, but the value of the FEV_1 was only significant on univariate analysis. Those patients with more homogenous or lower-lobe predominant emphysema fared worse; and lower exercise tolerance and age were also significant predictors. Of 609 patients in the medically treated cohort, 292 had died as of September 2005, after a median follow-up of only 3.9 years (12.7 deaths per 100 person-years).[56]

In keeping with a more multisystem approach to COPD, multifactorial scoring systems have been developed to provide a better indication to prognosis. The most established of these is the BODE score, incorporating *B*MI, the degree of airflow *O*bstruction, *D*yspnoea, and *E*xercise capacity.[57] The total score obtained correlates better than the FEV_1 with all-cause and respiratory mortality, and analysis of the NETT data shows that the change in a modified BODE score is of further short and intermediate term prognostic value.[58]

Acute Exacerbations

Acute exacerbations of COPD, as well as the obvious short-term impacts, have more far reaching consequences. There is subsequently a more rapid decline in FEV_1,[42] and exacerbations requiring hospital admission have a significant risk of mortality attached to them, with around 10% dying in hospital, and a 23%–43% 1-year mortality rate.[59,60] Mortality figures are even worse when the presentation is one of acute hypercapnic respiratory failure, with over half of those requiring invasive ventilation not surviving to discharge.[61] In those who survive their admission, 80% will be readmitted and approximately 50% will be dead at one year.[62] The increase in noninvasive ventilation facilities has improved immediate survival, and early pulmonary rehabilitation improves exercise capacity and health status at 3 months,[63] but exacerbations still represent one of the most dangerous aspects of the disease.

SUMMARY

The burden of disease attributable to emphysema is significant and growing, and is a leading cause of disability in middle and late life. There has traditionally been a rather nihilistic attitude toward emphysema and COPD, but with recent advances in the understanding of aetiological, pathophysiological, and prognostic mechanisms, and the increase in treatment options, this approach is no longer appropriate.

REFERENCES

1. Ruysch F. Observationum anatomico-chirurgicarum centuria. Amsterdam: Boom; 1691. Obs XIX, XX.
2. Baille M. The morbid anatomy of some of the most important parts of the human body. London: Johnson and Nicol; 1793.
3. Baille M. A series of engravings, accompanied with explanations which are intended to illustrate the morbid anatomy of the most important parts of the human body. London: W. Bulmer; 1799.
4. Laennec RTH. A treatise on the diseases of the chest and on mediate auscultation. Translated by J. Forbes. Fourth London edition. Philadelphia: Thomas and Co.; 1835.
5. Orsos F. Au uber das elastische Gerauust der normalen und der emphysematosen Lunge. Pathol Anat 1907;41:95–121.
6. Gough L. The pathological diagnosis of emphysema. Proc R Soc Med 1952;45(9):576–7.
7. Leopold JG, Gough J. The centrilobular form of hypertrophic emphysema and its relation to chronic bronchitis. Thorax 1957;12(3):219–35.
8. Fishman A, Martinez F, Naunheim K, et al. National Emphysema Treatment Trial Research Group. A randomized trial comparing lung-volume-reduction surgery with medical therapy for severe emphysema. N Engl J Med 2003;348:2059–73.
9. Strange C, Herth FJ, Kovitz KL, et al. VENT Study Group. Design of the Endobronchial Valve for Emphysema Palliation Trial (VENT): a non-surgical method of lung volume reduction. BMC Pulm Med 2007;7:10.
10. Wood DE, McKenna RJ Jr, Yusen RD, et al. A multicenter trial of an intrabronchial valve for treatment of severe emphysema. J Thorac Cardiovasc Surg 2007;133(1):65–73.
11. Rabe KF, Hurd S, Anzueto A, et al. Global initiative for chronic obstructive lung disease. Global strategy for the diagnosis, management, and prevention of chronic obstructive pulmonary disease: GOLD executive summary. Am J Respir Crit Care Med 2007;176(6):532–55.
12. Pauwels RA, Buist AS, Calverly PM, et al. GOLD Scientific Committee. Global strategy for the diagnosis, management, and prevention of chronic obstructive pulmonary disease. NHLBI/WHO Global Initiative for Chronic Obstructive Lung Disease (GOLD) workshop summary. Am J Respir Crit Care Med 2001;163(5):1256–76.
13. National Institute for Clinical Excellence (NICE). Chronic obstructive pulmonary disease: national clinical guideline for management of chronic obstructive pulmonary disease in adults in primary and secondary care. Thorax 2004;59(Suppl I).
14. World Health Organisation. Chronic obstructive pulmonary disease. Fact sheet No 315; May 2008. Available at: http://www.who.int/mediacentre/factsheets/fs315/en/.
15. Mannino DM, Gagnon RC, Petty TL, et al. Obstructive lung disease and low lung function in adults in the United States: data from the Nation Health and Nutrition Examination Survey 1988–1994. Arch Intern Med 2000;160:1683–9.
16. Soriano JB, Maier WC, Egger P, et al. Recent trends in physician diagnosed COPD in women and men in the UK. Thorax 2000;55:789–94.
17. Gupta PP, Agarwal D. A 24-year old man with persistent progressive breathlessness: early onset COPD. Prim Care Respir J 2007;16:387–90.
18. Fletcher C, Peto R. The natural history of chronic airflow obstruction. Br Med J 1977;1:1645–8.
19. Laurell C-B, Eriksson S. The electrophoretic α1-globulin pattern of serum in α1-antitrypsin deficiency. Scand J Clin Lab Invest 1963;15:132–40.
20. Laurell C-B. Studies on the transportation and metabolism of iron in the body. Acta Physiol Scand 1947;14:1–129.
21. Holmberg CG, Laurell C-B. Investigations in serum copper. II. Isolation of the copper containing protein, and a description of some of its properties. Acta Chem Scand 1948;2:550–6.
22. Laurell C-B, Nyman M. Studies on the serum haptoglobin level in hemoglobinemia and its influence on renal excretion of hemoglobin. Blood 1957;12:493–506.
23. Laurell C-B, Laurell H, Waldenström J. Glycoproteins in serum from patients with myeloma, macroglobulinemia and related conditions. Am J Med 1957;22:24–36.
24. de Serres FJ. Worldwide racial and ethnic distribution of alpha-1-antitrypsin deficiency: details of an analysis of published genetic epidemiological surveys. Chest 2002;122:1818–29.
25. Crystal RG, Brantly ML, Hubbard RC, et al. The alpha 1-antitrypsin gene and its mutations. Clinical consequences and strategies for therapy. Chest 1989;95(1):196–208.
26. Janus ED, Phillips NT, Carrell RW. Smoking, lung function, and alpha-1 antitrypsin deficiency. Lancet 1985;1(8421):152–4.
27. Hersh CP, Demeo DL, Lazarus R, et al. Genetic association analysis of functional impairment in chronic obstructive pulmonary disease. Am J Respir Crit Care Med 2006;173(9):977–84.
28. DeMeo DL, Hersh CP, Hoffman EA, et al. Genetic determinants of emphysema distribution in the

national emphysema treatment trial. Am J Respir Crit Care Med 2007;176(1):42–8.

29. Moshammer H, Hoek G, Luttman-Gibson H, et al. Parental smoking and lung function in children: an international study. Am J Respir Crit Care Med 2006;173(11):1255–63.

30. Shaheen SO, Barker DJ, Shiell AW, et al. The relationship between pneumonia in early childhood and impaired lung function in late adult life. Am J Respir Crit Care Med 1994;149(3 Pt 1):616–9.

31. Marossy AE, Strachen DP, Rudnicka AR, et al. Childhood chest illness and the rate of decline of adult lung function between ages 35 and 45 years. Am J Respir Crit Care Med 2007;175(4):355–9.

32. Howling SJ, Northway WH Jr, Hansell DM, et al. Pulmonary sequelae of bronchopulmonary dysplasia survivors: high-resolution CT findings. Am J Roentgenol 2000;174(5):1323–6.

33. Motley HL, Lang LP, Gordon B. Pulmonary emphysema and ventilation measurements in 100 anthracite coal miners with respiratory complaints. Am Rev Tuberc 1949;59(3):270–88.

34. Leigh J, Driscoll TR, Cole BD, et al. Quantitative relation between emphysema and lung mineral content in coalworkers. Occup Environ Med 1994;51:400–7.

35. Ulvestad B, Bakke B, Eduard W, et al. Cumulative exposure to dust causes accelerated decline in lung function in tunnel workers. Occup Environ Med 2001;58:663–9.

36. Becklake MR, Irwig L, Kielkowski D, et al. The predictors of emphysema in South African goldminers. Am Rev Respir Dis 1987;135:1234–41.

37. Hnizdo E, Sluis-Cremer GK, Abramowits JA. Emphysema type in relation to silica dust exposure in South African gold miners. Am Rev Respir Dis 1991;143: 1241–7.

38. Ozbay B, Uzun K, Arslan H, et al. Functional and radiological impairment in women highly exposed to indoor biomass fuels. Respirology 2001;6(3):255–8.

39. The World Health report: 2002: Reducing risks, promoting healthy life. Geneva (Switzerland) WHO; 2002.

40. Zhong N, Wang C, Yao W, et al. Prevalence of chronic obstructive pulmonary disease in China: a large, population-based survey. Am J Respir Crit Care Med 2007;176(8):753–60.

41. Fletcher C, Peto R, Tinker C, et al. The natural history of chronic bronchitis and emphysema. Toronto. New York: Oxford University Press; 1976.

42. Donaldson GC, Seemungal TAR, Bhomik A, et al. Relationship between exacerbation frequency and lung function decline in chronic obstructive pulmonary disease. Thorax 2002;57:847–52.

43. Wilkinson TMA, Patel IS, Wilks M, et al. Airway bacterial load and FEV_1 decline in patients with chronic obstructive lung disease. Am J Respir Crit Care Med 2003;167:1090–5.

44. Thabut G, Dauriat G, Stern JB, et al. Pulmonary hemodynamics in advanced COPD candidates for lung volume reduction surgery or lung transplantation. Chest 2005;127:1531–6.

45. Eddahibi S, Chaouat A, Morrell N, et al. Polymorphism of the serotonin transporter gene and pulmonary hypertension in chronic obstructive pulmonary disease. Circulation 2003;108:1839–44.

46. Swallow EB, Reyes D, Hopkinson NS, et al. Quadriceps strength predicts mortality in patients with moderate to severe chronic obstructive pulmonary disease. Thorax 2007;62(2):115–20.

47. Hopkinson NS, Nickol AH, Payne J, et al. Angiotensin converting enzyme genotype and strength in chronic obstructive pulmonary disease. Am J Respir Crit Care Med 2004;170(4):395–9.

48. Hopkinson NS, Li KW, Kehoe A, et al. Vitamin D receptor genotypes influence quadriceps strength in chronic obstructive pulmonary disease. Am J Clin Nutr 2008;87(2):385–90.

49. Kohn HN. Zur Histologie des indurirenden fibrinösen Pneumonia. Münch Med Woch 1893;40:42–5.

50. Terry PB, Traystman RJ, Newball HH, et al. Collateral ventilation in man. N Engl J Med 1978;298(1): 10–5.

51. Cormier Y, Atton L, Sériès F. Influence of lung volume hysteresis on collateral resistance in intact dogs. Lung 1993;171(1):43–51.

52. Fletcher CM, Peto R, Tinker CM, et al. The natural history of chronic bronchitis and emphysema. An eight year study of early chronic obstructive lung disease in working men in London. Oxford (UK): Oxford University Press; 1976.

53. Monsó E, Izquierdo J, Alonson J, et al. Quality of life in severe chronic obstructive pulmonary disease: correlation with lung and muscle function. Respir Med 1998;92(2):221–7.

54. Spencer S, Calverley PM, Sherwood Burge P, et al. Health status deterioration in patients with chronic obstructive pulmonary disease. Am J Respir Crit Care Med 2001;163(1):122–8.

55. Naunheim KS, Wood DE, Mohsenifah S, et al. Long-term follow-up of patients receiving lung-volume-reduction surgery versus medical therapy for severe emphysema by the National Emphysema Treatment Trial Research Group. Ann Thorac Surg 2006;82: 431–43.

56. Martinez FJ, Foster G, Curtis JL, et al. Predictors of mortality in patients with severe emphysema and severe airflow obstruction. Am J Respir Crit Care Med 2006;173(12):1326–34.

57. Celli BR, Cote CG, Marin JM, et al. The body-mass index, airflow obstruction, dyspnea, and exercise capacity index in chronic obstructive pulmonary disease. N Engl J Med 2004;350(10):1005–12.

58. Martinez FJ, Han MK, Andrei AC, et al. Longitudinal changes in the Bode index predicts mortality in

severe emphysema. Am J Respir Crit Care Med 2008;178:491–9.

59. Connors AF Jr, Dawson NV, Thomas C, et al. Outcomes following acute exacerbation of severe chronic obstructive lung disease. The SUPPORT investigators (Study to Understand Prognoses and Preferences for Outcomes and Risks of Treatments). Am J Respir Crit Care Med 1999;154(4 pt 1):959–67.

60. Kaplan RM, Ries AL, Reilly J, et al. Measurement of health-related quality of life in the national emphysema treatment trial. Chest 2004;126:781–9.

61. Ucgun I, Metinas M, Moral H, et al. Predictors of hospital outcome and intubation in COPD patients admitted to the respiratory ICU for acute hypercapnic respiratory failure. Respir Med 2006;100(1): 66–74.

62. Chu CM, Chan VL, Lin AW, et al. Readmission rates and life threatening events in COPD survivors treated with non-invasive ventilation for acute hypercapnic respiratory failure. Thorax 2004;59(12): 1020–5.

63. Man WD, Polkey MI, Donaldson N, et al. Community pulmonary rehabilitation after hospitalisation for acute exacerbations of chronic obstructive pulmonary disease: randomised controlled study. BMJ 2004;329(7476):1209–11.

Update on Radiology of Emphysema and Therapeutic Implications

Jonathan G. Goldin, MD, PhD*, Fereidoun Abtin, MD

KEYWORDS

• Emphysema • CT • Clinical trials • Quantitation • Function

Emphysema is characterized on CT by the presence of areas of abnormally low attenuation.[1,2] CT, and in particular volumetric acquired high resolution CT (HRCT, 06–2 mm), is excellent for detecting the presence of and for demonstrating the pattern, distribution, and extent of emphysema. Recently the accepted standard of using thick-section CT (5–10 mm) has been shown to be less reliable than high-resolution volume acquisition CT images.[3,4] Emphysema is a heterogeneous process that varies widely in pattern and distribution from one subject to another, which can be evaluated from full chest volumetric data.

CT ACQUISITION PROTOCOLS

With modern multislice techniques the lungs can be scanned easily in a single breath hold by patients who have even moderately severe emphysema. Controlling for lung volume is important for quantitative assessment of emphysema, especially on serial studies taken to evaluate an intervention.[5] There is ongoing debate as to whether reproducibility of scan volumes requires integrated respiratory gating control of the scanner or whether this can be achieved without spirometric control.[6–8] There is also the logistic issue that respiratory gating is not easily available. In general, with careful attention to breathing instructions imaging at suspended volumes is good enough.[8]

Scans are usually acquired at suspended full inspiration, which has been reported to have a greater consistency in the volume of scans than those performed at end expiration.[9–11] Density measures at end expiration have been shown to have a good correlation between pixels less than -950 Hounsfield units (HU) ($r = 0.55$) and macroscopic morphometric evidence for emphysema.[12] Expiratory scans can, however, reveal air trapping in patients who have small airways obstruction even when inspiratory scans appear normal.[13,14] Overall lung density can vary by as much as 80 to 100 HU from full inspiration to end expiration.[15,16] Several investigators have reported that expiratory scans have shown higher correlation with pulmonary function tests using density masks calculated on expiratory scans.[17,18] In recent work, intermediate densities of -900 to -950 had a correlation coefficient as high as -0.86 between the ratio of these pixels on inspiration and expiration and the pulmonary function tests.[19] Others have found no advantage in expiratory scans but have demonstrated greater consistency in the volume of scans made at total lung capacity compared with those done at lower volumes.

VISUAL ASSESSMENT

It has been well established that the sensitivity in the detection and the accuracy of assessing severity of emphysema is excellent.[1–6,8,20,21] The extent of emphysema can be estimated subjectively by visual inspection.[22,23] The correlation between in vivo CT emphysema score and the

Department of Radiology, Thoracic Imaging Research Group, David Geffen School of Medicine at UCLA, 924 Westwood Boulevard, Suite #650, Los Angeles, CA 90024, USA
* Corresponding author.
E-mail address: jgoldin@mednet.ucla.edu (J.G. Goldin).

Thorac Surg Clin 19 (2009) 159–167
doi:10.1016/j.thorsurg.2009.04.006
1547-4127/09/$ – see front matter © 2009 Elsevier Inc. All rights reserved.

pathologic grade is reported to be between 0.7 and 0.9, although several groups have reported that CT scans can miss early emphysema.[3,4,21,24–26] Visual scoring studies have for the most part shown good agreement between expert readers for assessment of the presence and extent of emphysema,[3,27,28] and good correlation between the subjective and objective analysis of emphysema.[27]

COMPUTER-AIDED ASSESSMENT

There is increasing interest in the role of computer-based algorithms to detect and score emphysema severity and even to classify the different patterns.[27,29–38] One of the attributes of CT is that it is in its fundamental design a densitometer, and lung absorbs X-rays in direct correlation to the density of the lung tissue present.[39] Although the normal human lung has a symmetric distribution of X-ray attenuation values around a mean of approximately −800 HU, reduction in the quantity of tissue in the lung causes changes in the shape of this distribution and the percentage of lung voxels with a given X-ray attenuation value. A quantitative CT assessment of the lung not only provides spatial information about larger structures within the lung but, through densitometry, inferences about the microstructure of the tissue and airspace can be drawn. The frequency distribution of attenuation values (**Fig. 1**) and derived measures from this distribution are often used through the entire lung, lobe, segment, or other region of interest to measure the amount of emphysema.[35–38]

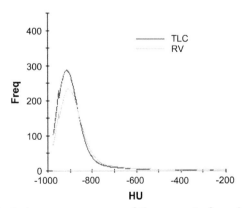

Fig. 1. A common measure of the amount of emphysema is to plot the frequency distribution of pixel density measures (HU) and then to either use a fixed threshold (eg, less than −950 HU) or a given percentile measure (eg, lowest 15th centile) or to calculate the area under the curve.

There are several measures that can be derived from this frequency distribution. Mean lung density (MLD) is calculated by averaging the density of all pixels in the image that represent the entire lung. It has been correlated positively with lung function tests.[29,39–41] The percentile point is defined as the cutoff density value in HU, for which a predetermined percentage of all voxels has a lower value and, as with MLD, is also influenced by density changes in all lung structures.[42,43] Only the fifth percentile point has been correlated with pathology[30] and lung function tests,[44] although in the assessment of emphysema progression there is similar sensitivity between the 10th, 15th, and 20th percentile.[5,30,34] The voxel index (VI), also referred to as Density Mask after the software program developed by General Electric Medical Systems (Milwaukee, Wisconsin), or the "relative area," is defined as the proportional area under the curve of the histogram below a predetermined threshold. It is not influenced by changes in the attenuation value of voxels that remain beyond the designated threshold. Different thresholds have been applied and validated by comparative studies using pathologic standards[12,21,27,44–46] and physiology.[17,27,31,32,46–49] Muller and colleagues[27] showed that on conventional 10-mm thick sections, a threshold of −910 HU, which highlights all pixels with attenuation values less than −910, correlates best with the extent of emphysema. Similarly good results using −910 HU have been reported by others.[33] Gevenois and colleagues[21,46] have shown that, using 1-mm sections, the optimal threshold for HRCT images when compared with morphometric data is −950 HU.

CT attenuation values are recognized to depend on scanner type, model, object positioning within the scanner gantry, and various physical factors (eg, kilovoltage, current-time product, slice thickness, and reconstruction algorithm).[47–52] Lung density also depends on inspiratory level, and the volume of air in the lungs can be used to adjust lung density for the inspiratory level. When analyzing trends in longitudinal data there is debate as to whether the density measure should be corrected for lung because the total lung volume of a subject may vary significantly from one examination to the next.[5] This kind of noise reduction may be less important in cross-sectional studies, such as the one by Dawkins and colleagues,[53] and it may even introduce new errors. An increase in total lung volume is an inherent part of the emphysematous process and, by eliminating that aspect of the disease, volume adjustment may in fact weaken the correlation between CT lung density and other measures of disease severity (Goldin, unpublished data, 2009). Adjustment of lung density for lung volume thus remains an area of active debate. Perhaps a better strategy is to ensure good reproducibility of lung volume at which scans are obtained akin to guidelines in the lung function laboratory.[54] **Fig. 2** demonstrates that good reproducibility of density scores can be achieved in multicenter studies using this approach.

The development of sophisticated computer programs, coupled with spiral CT scanners, now allows practical quantitative three-dimensional (3D) CT assessment of either select regions or entire lung volumes in a single breath-hold period.[36–38] Using 5 mm and 7 mm collimation with a pitch of 1.5, Park and colleagues[32] found good correlation between 3D assessment of both mean lung attenuation values and frequency distribution histograms of whole lungs compared with routine two-dimensional analysis ($r = 0.98–0.99$) and visual scoring ($r = 0.74–0.82$), respectively. Coxson and colleagues[33] developed prediction equations that allow quantification of lung surface area and lung surface-to-volume ratio and surface area. They showed that mild emphysema is associated with an increase in lung volume and a reduction in surface-to-volume ratio, whereas surface area and tissue weight are only decreased with severe disease. The CT-predicted surface-to-volume ratio correlated well with the histologic findings;[55] it is becoming increasingly well known that quantifying the extent of the disease is only part of the solution. Other studies have suggested that measures of emphysematous hole size[56] and distribution may be important, particularly in lung volume reduction surgery (LVRS).[57]

RELATIONSHIP BETWEEN CT AND FUNCTIONAL ASSESSMENT OF EMPHYSEMA

It has been established that the sensitivity of HRCT in detecting early emphysematous change is higher than that of pulmonary function tests.[20,58,59]

Patients who have predominantly upper-lobe emphysema and normal lower lobes as identified by HRCT have near normal pulmonary function tests compared with those who have predominantly lower-lobe emphysema,[58] which implies that the anatomic site of the emphysema determines the degree of impairment of lung function. Chest CT, on the other hand, focuses on anatomic changes, and has the potential to evaluate tissue changes at the local and regional level.[60–63] CT may therefore provide the ability to detect subtle, regional changes that are not identifiable by pulmonary function tests.[26] Longitudinal studies indicate that densitometric indices relate to the decline in FEV_1[64] but in addition are a more sensitive measure of emphysema progression than pulmonary function tests and health status.[65–68] Quantitative measures derived from CT are being increasingly evaluated as potential biomarker predictive of treatment outcome.[69]

In addition to quantitation of structural damage at static lung volumes, analysis of the rate of change in HU during a forced vital capacity maneuver plotted against time can give additional functional information. The plot of the change in CT density of lung versus time (HU/T) for normal lungs demonstrates maximum flow, and increase in lung attenuation occurs within the first 2 to 4 seconds of forced expiration that parallels the volume time curve. In patients who have obstructed airflow, such as severe emphysema, airflow is considerably decreased and there is minimal change in lung attenuation over time, resulting in marked flattening of the HU/T curve. Despite similar visually apparent extent of structural damage because of emphysema, HU/T and lung attenuation curve curves can show marked differences in airflow and air trapping, offering further insights into the pathophysiology of emphysema. This insight can also be useful in assessing split lung function in patients who have emphysema who have undergone single lung

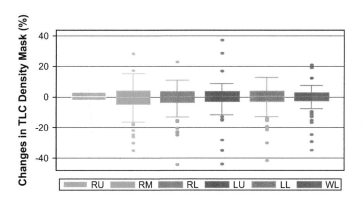

Fig. 2. The density scores, in this case the percentage of pixels less than −910 HU, from thick-section volumetric CT acquired at multiple sites in a multicenter study show good reproducibly for each lobe in a control group of subjects scanned on the same machine using a standardized breath hold and imaging protocol at baseline and 6 months' follow-up.

transplantation. A classic early dynamic collapse pattern with late terminal flow is noted on spirometry in these patients. Although at first believed to be attributable to the dynamic collapse of the anastomotic lung, the HU/T analysis performed during a forced expiration maneuver demonstrates that the terminal phase is, in fact, most likely due to the slow flow from the native obstructed lung where flow is seen to occur after complete emptying of the transplant lung.[70] The differential airflow of the transplant lung can be easily assessed independently of the native lung in these patients. This procedure can be useful in the detection of early anastomotic complications leading to obstruction (**Fig. 3**).[71]

CT IN EMPHYSEMA TREATMENT PLANNING AND EFFICACY

Research into the therapeutic options for patients who have emphysema has expanded greatly in this decade. The goal of most of the interventions is to decrease the volume of the lobe most severely affected by emphysema allowing for the less severely affected lobes to expand and improve ventilation. There are several approaches, including bronchoscopic lung volume reduction using one-way valves,[72,73] use of airway sealants, use of endobronchial spigots and plugs,[74] or endobronchial bypass methods allowing for the trapped air to escape by way of an alternative route through bronchial stents and fenestrations.[75] These treatment options require appropriate CT targeting of a selected lobe or lobes and target airways to obtain a successful response, and investigations are directed toward optimization of the targeting. CT scan is used in pretreatment planning to select patients and plan treatment strategy and posttreatment to confirm correct

deployment of devices and assess treatment response (**Fig. 4**).

PATTERN AND DISTRIBUTION OF EMPHYSEMA IN TREATMENT PLANNING

The extent and lobar distribution of emphysema and its influence on treatment outcome and survival was first shown in the National Emphysema Treatment Trial (NETT).[76] LVRS did yield a survival advantage for patients who had predominantly upper-lobe emphysema and low baseline exercise capacity.[77] Although the lobar selection in NETT was suboptimal and was based on approximate distribution and quantitation of emphysema and visual scoring of noncontiguous image data sets, the influence of lobar distribution and heterogeneity on treatment outcome and the need for correct and reproducible quantitation of emphysema is evident.[76,77] CT scan has also proved to be an accurate and reproducible modality for evaluation of lung volume and function, particularly while evaluating total lung capacity and RV, allowing for detection of a subgroup of patients benefiting from each of the available interventions.[36]

The extent and distribution of emphysema in the lung is usually quantitated and scored using Goddard scale.[78] Heterogeneous emphysema as detailed by difference in two adjacent lobes of more that 25% or difference of 1 on the Goddard scale is the selection criteria for LVRS and endobronchial procedures, particularly with endobronchial valves and plugs. Some require visual scoring but some investigators require computer aided diagnosis-automated CT quantitation and lobar segmentation of emphysema.[73] Either method requires accurate and reproducible CT scans. The advantage of lobar segmentation of emphysema lies in the ability to obtain

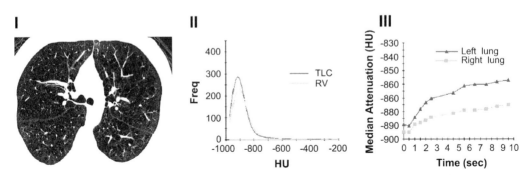

Fig. 3. Axial section from a patient who had emphysema demonstrating that both lungs have the same amount of emphysema destruction but almost no difference in overall air trapping and density at residual volume compared with total lung capacity. The rate of emptying as measured by the rate of change of lung density over time (HU/T) demonstrates a marked difference in function between the relatively rapid emptying left lung and the slow emptying of the right lung.

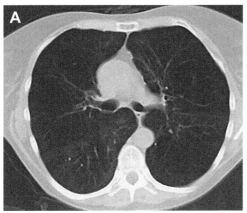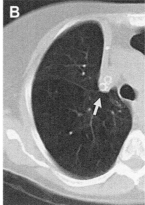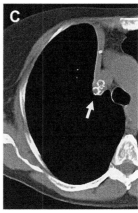

Fig. 4. CT scan screening for quantitation of emphysema for endobronchial valve (EBV) therapy. Pre-treatment screening CT scan (*A*) in lung window at the level of right upper lobe (RUL) bronchus shows predominantly upper lobe emphysema with patent RUL bronchus. CT scan in lung (*B*) and soft tissue (*C*) window following EBV placement shows the valves (*white arrow*) in upper-lobe segmental airways with lobar occlusion and complete collapse of right upper lobe.

reproducible data without any inter- or intra-reader variation and the ability to compare the baseline to follow-up CT scan for progression and treatment response.

Homogenous emphysema is being targeted for treatment by endobronchial fenestration and stents. Homogenous emphysema is described as score of 1 or less between the lobes. Placement of bronchial stents takes advantage of the extensive collateral ventilation present in emphysematous lungs to provide improvement in expiratory flow and respiratory mechanics.[75] The distribution of disease and air trapping demonstrated by the inability to expire adequate volumes and lack of decrease in lobar volume during RV is evaluated with CT scan and used for target lobe selection.[74,79] CT scan is also used for detection of bullous disease before placement of stents. Large bullae are contraindicated because there is increased chance of pneumothorax.

FISSURE INTEGRITY AND COLLATERAL FLOW

In addition to pattern of distribution, target lobe selection may also require other imaging features to be assessed. For some of the devices being assess a closed system is required to facilitate treatment efficacy. The effects of collateral flow are particularly accentuated in patients who have emphysema.[80,81] Abtin and colleagues[81,82] in a recent study suggested that fissure integrity may be an important imaging biomarker of collateral flow between lobes. In this study fissure integrity was assessed and scored on thin-section full-volume CT data acquired in the VENT study.[73] All CT scan images were acquired with less than

1.25 mm collimation and viewed in axial, sagittal, and coronal planes. The integrity of the fissure completeness referred to as fissure integrity score (FIS) was scored on scale of 0 to 4 as follows: 4, complete fissure; 3, more than 90% of fissure present; 2, 10%–90% of fissure present; 1, less than 10% of fissure present; and 0, absent fissures.[81,82] The scoring is performed on CT scan images obtained on thin-slice thickness less than 1.25 mm to allow accurate analysis of fissures and multiplanar reconstruction (**Fig. 5**). Presence of partial fissures corresponding to FIS equal to or less than 3, in this study, was correlated with a significant reduction in demonstrated target lobe atelectasis. The investigators concluded that an incomplete fissure allowed for collateral flow to drift between lobes to circulate distal to the occluded target lobe bronchus undermining the treatment response.

AIRWAY ANATOMY, VARIANCE, AND SAFETY SCORE

CT scan plays a vital role in selection of the bronchial region safe for fenestration and drug-eluting stent placement. Anatomically these stents are placed centrally and close to the hilum, because of the limited ability of bronchoscopes to extend into airways smaller than 5 mm and more peripherally, thereby increasing the possibility of injury to pulmonary vessels. Ultrasound guidance probe (Broncus Technologies Inc., Mountain View, California) is used to identify the locations of the adjacent vessels before deployment of the radioablation catheter.[74,75] For the ultrasound probes to be in approximate close location, CT

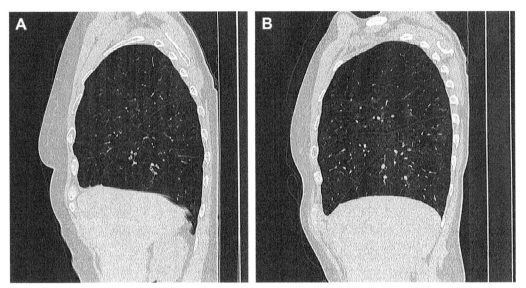

Fig. 5. Sagittal reconstruction through the mid right hemithorax of two patients who had emphysema. (*A*) Relatively homogenous distribution through all segments is seen. The right minor fissure is only seen through the proximal extent and is an example of an incomplete fissure (fissure integrity score [FIS] = 2). (*B*) Heterogeneous pattern of emphysema with upper lobe predominance. The right horizontal and oblique fissures were intact throughout their extent (FIS = 4 for both).

guidance and bronchial mapping are performed. In addition, Ochs and colleagues[83] have developed semiautomated image processing techniques to aid the visual assessment of the airways. This assessment allows prebronchoscopy virtual mapping and assessment of pretreatment airway sites for a large number of variances in bronchial anatomy and the number and size of the valves or extent of plugs needed. The software developed allows 3D mapping of each bronchial segment and adjacent vital structures and development of safety score. Based on the CT data the program also allows for detection of the distance required by the bronchoscope to reach a safe zone and the percentage diameter of bronchus free of vascular margins and the vessel-free surface, in turn allowing safer placement of stents.

CT also helps detection and proximity of other vital structures, including the aorta, heart, and fissures. The aorta is found usually in close proximity to the superior segment of the left lower lobe. Both the oblique fissures are in close proximity to anterior and anteromedial segmental bronchi of the right and left lower lobes, respectively. Placement of stents within the fissures causes prolonged pneumothorax and pneumomediastinum. In addition to safety evaluation and scoring, CT allows evaluation of bronchial diameter and luminal diameter, both of which are necessary information before placement of stents.

RADIATION DOSE CONSIDERATIONS

It is important to keep in mind the radiation burden to the subject imparted by CT scans. The effective radiation dose to the chest for a volume acquisition CT examination has been estimated to be 5 to 8 mSv. Conventional examinations are done with an mAs setting of 180 to 240, but with a kilovolt peak (kVp) of 120 to 140; doses of 100 mAs are common in chest screening, and 20 to 40 mAs can be used for emphysema quantification, representing a 6- to 10-fold dose reduction.[84,85] The noise level of the image, and hence the variance of the density or the blurriness of the structures, varies with the dose. This variation may have limited effect on the density mask score, but there is enough difference that some investigators avoid automatic dose reduction, which is available on newer machines. Madani and colleagues[55] showed there is no reason that low-dose CT scans cannot be used; in fact, they should be used for serial measurements of emphysema, but the CT parameters must not be changed between scans.

In summary, full-volume thin-section thoracic CT is an important part of the pre- and posttreatment assessment of patients who have emphysema. Quantitative CT analysis of lung density is a powerful technique to assess emphysema allowing for objective quantification, which is a more consistent assessment of disease extent than subjective analysis. These quantitative measurements on CT scanning can be affected by several variables, including patient size, depth of inspiration, type of CT scanner used, collimation, and the reconstruction algorithm. Emerging treatments require appropriate CT targeting of a selected lobe or lobes and target airways to obtain a successful response, and investigations are directed at optimization of the targeting. CT scan is used in both pretreatment planning to select patients and plan treatment strategy and posttreatment to confirm correct deployment of devices and assess treatment response.

REFERENCES

1. Hruban RH, Meziane MA, Zerhouni EA, et al. High resolution computed tomography of inflation fixed lungs: pathologic-radiologic correlation of centrilobular emphysema. Am Rev Respir Dis 1987;136: 935–40.

2. Webb WR, Stein MG, Finkbeiner WE, et al. Normal and diseased isolated lungs: high-resolution CT. Radiology 1988;166:81–7.

3. Miller RR, Müller NL, Vedal S, et al. Limitations of computed tomography in the assessment of emphysema. Am Rev Respir Dis 1989;139:980–3.

4. Kuwano K, Matsuba K, Ikeda T, et al. The diagnosis of mild emphysema: correlation of computed tomography and pathology scores. Am Rev Respir Dis 1990;141:169–78.

5. Dirksen A, Friis M, Olesen KP, et al. Progress of emphysema in severe alpha 1-antitrypsin deficiency as assessed by annual CT. Acta Radiol 1997;38: 826–32.

6. Kauczor HU, Hast J, Heussel CP, et al. CT attenuation of paired HRCT scans obtained at full inspiratory/expiratory position: comparison with pulmonary function tests. Eur Radiol 2002;12: 2757–63.

7. Hoffman EA, McLennan G. Assessment of the pulmonary structure-function relationship and clinical outcomes measures: quantitative volumetric CT of the lung. Acad Radiol 1997;4:758–76.

8. Gierada DS, Yusen RD, Pilgram TK, et al. Repeatability of quantitative CT indexes of emphysema in patients evaluated for lung volume reduction surgery. Radiology 2001;220:448–54.

9. Robinson PJ, Kreel L. Pulmonary tissue attenuation with computed tomography: comparison of inspiration and expiration scans. J Comput Assist Tomogr 1979;3:740–8.

10. Lamers RJ, Kemerink GJ, Drent M, et al. Reproducibility of spirometrically controlled CT lung densitometry in a clinical setting. Eur Respir J 1998;11:942–5.

11. Siegelman S. Pulmonary system: practical approaches to pulmonary diagnosis. New York: Grune and Stratton; 1979.

12. Gevenois PA, De Vuyst P, Sy M, et al. Pulmonary emphysema: quantitative CT during expiration. Radiology 1996;199:825–9.

13. Stern EJ, Frank MS. Small-airway diseases of the lungs: findings at expiratory CT. AJR Am J Roentgenol 1994;163:37–41.

14. Lee KW, Chung SY, Yang I, et al. Correlation of aging and smoking with air trapping at thin-section CT of the lung in asymptomatic subjects. Radiology 2000;214:831–6.

15. Van Dyk J, Keane TJ, Rider WD. Lung density as measured by computerized tomography: implications for radiotherapy. Int J Radiat Oncol Biol Phys 1982;8:1363–72.

16. Wegener OH, Koeppe P, Oeser H. Measurement of lung density by computed tomography. J Comput Assist Tomogr 1978;2:263–73.

17. Camiciottoli G, Bartolucci M, Maluccio NM, et al. Spirometrically gated high-resolution CT findings in COPD: lung attenuation versus lung function and dyspnea severity. Chest 2006;129:558–64.

18. Zaporozhan J, Ley S, Eberhardt R, et al. Paired inspiratory/expiratory volumetric thin-slice CT scan for emphysema analysis: comparison of different quantitative evaluations and pulmonary function test. Chest 2005;128:3212–20.

19. Matsuoka S, Kurihara Y, Yagihashi K, et al. Quantitative assessment of peripheral airway obstruction on paired expiratory/inspiratory thin-section computed tomography in chronic obstructive pulmonary disease with emphysema. J Comput Assist Tomogr 2007;31:384–9.

20. Thurlbeck WM, Müller NL. Emphysema: definition, imaging, and quantification. AJR Am J Roentgenol 1994;163:1017–25.

21. Gevenois PA, de Maertelaer V, De Vuyst P, et al. Comparison of computed density and macroscopic morphometry in pulmonary emphysema. Am J Respir Crit Care Med 1995;152:653–7.

22. Sakai F, Gamsu G, Im JG, et al. Pulmonary function abnormalities in patients with CT-determined emphysema. J Comput Assist Tomogr 1987;11:963–8.

23. Nishimura K, Murata K, Yamagishi M, et al. Comparison of different computed tomography scanning methods for quantifying emphysema. J Thorac Imaging 1998;13:193–8.

24. Spouge D, Mayo JR, Cardoso W, et al. Panacinar emphysema: CT and pathologic correlation. J Comput Assist Tomogr 1993;17:710–3.

25. Bergin CJ, Müller NL, Miller RR. CT in the qualitative assessment of emphysema. J Thorac Imaging 1986; 1:94–103.

26. Remy-Jardin M, Remy J, Gosselin B, et al. Sliding thin slab, minimum intensity projection technique in

the diagnosis of emphysema: histopathologic-CT correlation. Radiology 1996;200:665–71.

27. Muller NL, Staples CA, Miller RR, et al. "Density mask." An objective method to quantitate emphysema using computed tomography. Chest 1988;94:782–7.

28. Gelb AF, Zamel N, Hogg JC, et al. Pseudophysiologic emphysema resulting from small-airways disease. Am J Respir Crit Care Med 1998;158:815–9.

29. Hayhurst MD, Flenley DC, McLean A, et al. Diagnosis of pulmonary emphysema by computerized tomography. Lancet 1984;2:320–2.

30. Gould GA, Macnee W, McLean A, et al. CT measurements of lung density in life can quantitate distal airspace enlargement: an essential defining feature of human emphysema. Am Rev Respir Dis 1988; 137:380–92.

31. Gevenois PA, Yernault JC. Can computed tomography quantify pulmonary emphysema? Eur Respir J 1995;8:843–8.

32. Park KJ, Bergin CJ, Clausen JL. Quantitation of emphysema with three-dimensional CT densitometry: comparison with two-dimensional analysis, visual emphysema scores, and pulmonary function test results. Radiology 1999;211:541–7.

33. Coxson HO, Rogers RM, Whittall KP, et al. A quantification of lung surface area in emphysema using computed tomography. Am J Respir Crit Care Med 1999;159:851–6.

34. Bae KT, Slone RM, Gierada DS, et al. Patients with emphysema: quantitative CT analysis before and after lung volume reduction surgery. Work in progress. Radiology 1997;203:705–14.

35. Zagers H, Vrooman HA, Aarts NJ, et al. Assessment of the progression of emphysema by quantitative analysis of spirometrically gated computed tomography images. Invest Radiol 1996;31:761–7.

36. Brown MS, McNitt-Gray MF, Goldin JG, et al. Automated measurement of single and total lung volume from CT. J Comput Assist Tomogr 1999;23(4):632–40.

37. Kauczor HU, Heussel CP, Fischer B, et al. Assessment of lung volumes using helical CT at inspiration and expiration: comparison with pulmonary function tests. AJR Am J Roentgenol 1998;171:1091–5.

38. Mergo PJ, Williams WF, Gonzalez-Rothi R, et al. Three-dimensional volumetric assessment of abnormally low-attenuation of the lung from routine helical CT: inspiratory and expiratory quantification. AJR Am J Roentgenol 1998;170:1355–60.

39. Hedlund LW, Vock P, Effmann EL. Evaluating lung density by computed tomography. Semin Respir Med 1983;5:76–87.

40. Haraguchi M, Shimura S, Hida W, et al. Pulmonary function and regional distribution of emphysema as determined by high-resolution computed tomography. Respiration 1998;65:125–9.

41. Heremans A, Verschakelen JA, Van Fraeyenhoven L, et al. Measurement of lung density by means of quantitative CT scanning. A study of correlations with pulmonary function tests. Chest 1992;102:805–11.

42. Hartley PG, Galvin JR, Hunninghake GW, et al. High-resolution CT-derived measures of lung density are valid indexes of interstitial lung disease. J Appl Physiol 1994;76:271–7.

43. Rienmuller RK, Behr J, Kalender WA, et al. Standardized quantitative high resolution CT in lung diseases. J Comput Assist Tomogr 1991;15:742–9.

44. Gould GA, Redpath AT, Ryan M, et al. Lung CT density correlates with measurements of airflow limitation and the diffusing capacity. Eur Respir J 1991;4:141–6.

45. Bankier AA, De Maertelaer V, Keyzer C, et al. Pulmonary emphysema: subjective visual grading versus objective quantification with macroscopic morphometry and thin-section CT densitometry. Radiology 1999;211:851–8.

46. Gevenois PA, De Vuyst P, De Maertelaer V, et al. Comparison of computed density and microscopic morphometry in pulmonary emphysema. Am J Respir Crit Care Med 1996;154:187–92.

47. Kemerink GJ, Lamers RJ, Thelissen GR, et al. CT densitometry of the lungs: scanner performance. J Comput Assist Tomogr 1996;20:24–33.

48. Levi C, Gray JE, McCullough EC, et al. The unreliability of CT numbers as absolute values. AJR Am J Roentgenol 1982;139:443–7.

49. Kemerink GJ, Lamers RJ, Thelissen GR, et al. Scanner conformity in CT densitometry of the lungs. Radiology 1995;197:749–52.

50. Kemerink GJ, Kruize HH, Lamers RJ, et al. CT lung densitometry: dependence of CT number histograms on sample volume and consequences for scan protocol comparability. J Comput Assist Tomogr 1997;21:948–54.

51. McCullough EC. Specifying and evaluating the performance of computed tomography (CT) scanners. Med Phys 1980;7:291–6.

52. Boedeker KL, McNitt-Gray MF, Rogers SR, et al. Emphysema: effect of reconstruction algorithm on CT imaging measures. Radiology 2004;232: 295–301.

53. Dawkins PA, Dowson LJ, Guest PJ, et al. Predictors of mortality in α1-antitrypsin deficiency. Thorax 2003; 58:1020–6.

54. Miller MR, Crapo R, Hankinson J, et al. General consideration for lung function testing. Eur Respir J 2005;26:153–61.

55. Madani A, De Maertelaer V, Zanen J, et al. Pulmonary emphysema: radiation dose and section thickness at multidetector CT quantification – comparison with macroscopic and microscopic morphometry. Radiology 2007;243:250–7.

56. Mishima M, Hirai T, Itoh H, et al. Complexity of terminal airspace geometry assessed by lung computed tomography in normal subjects and patients with chronic obstructive pulmonary

disease. Proc Natl Acad Sci U S A 1999;96: 8829–34.

57. Coxson HO, Whittall KP, Nakano Y, et al. Selection of patients for lung volume reduction surgery using a power law analysis of the computed tomographic scan. Thorax 2003;58:510–4.

58. Gurney JW, Jones KK, Robbins RA, et al. Regional distribution of emphysema: correlation of high-resolution CT with pulmonary function tests in unselected smokers. Radiology 1992;183:457–63.

59. Klein JS, Gamsu G, Webb WR, et al. High-resolution CT diagnosis of emphysema in symptomatic patients with normal chest radiographs and isolated low diffusing capacity. Radiology 1992;182: 817–21.

60. Murata K, Itoh H, Todo G, et al. Centrilobular lesions of the lung: demonstration by high-resolution CT and pathologic correlation. Radiology 1986;161:641–5.

61. Murata K, Khan A, Herman PG. Pulmonary parenchymal disease: evaluation with high-resolution CT. Radiology 1989;170:629–35.

62. Guest PJ, Hansell DM. High resolution computed tomography (HRCT) in emphysema associated with alpha-1-antitrypsin deficiency. Clin Radiol 1992;45:260–6.

63. Brown MS, McNitt-Gray MF, Goldin JG, et al. Method for segmenting chest CT image data using an anatomical model: preliminary results. IEEE Trans Med Imaging 1997;16:828–39.

64. Parr DG, Stoel BC, Stolk J, et al. Validation of computed tomographic lung densitometry for monitoring emphysema in α1-antitrypsin deficiency. Thorax 2006;61:485–90.

65. Biernacki W, Ryan M, MacNee, et al. Can the quantitative CT scan detect progression of emphysema? Am Rev Respir Dis 1989;131:A120.

66. Dirksen A, Dijkman JH, Madsen F, et al. A randomized clinical trial of α1-antitrypsin augmentation therapy. Am J Respir Crit Care Med 1999;160:1468–72.

67. Dowson LJ, Guest PJ, Stockley RA, et al. Longitudinal changes in physiological, radiological, and health status measurements in α1-antitrypsin deficiency and factors associated with decline. Am J Respir Crit Care Med 2001;164:1805–9.

68. Soejima K, Yamaguchi K, Kohda E, et al. Longitudinal follow-up study of smoking-induced lung density changes by high-resolution computed tomography. Am J Respir Crit Care Med 2000;161:1264–73.

69. Long FR, Williams RS, Castile RG. Inspiratory and expiratory CT lung density in infants and young children. Pediatr Radiol 2005;35:677–83.

70. Szold O, Levine MS, Goldin JG, et al. Late expiratory plateau patients in post-single lung transplant patients with emphysema. Am J Respir Crit Care Med 1995;151(4):A85.

71. Levine MS, Shpiner RB, Martin K, et al. Clinical evaluation of stent placement in patients with persistent dyspnea in post single lung transplant (SLT). Am J Respir Crit Care Med 1997;155(4):A275.

72. Yim AP, Hwong TM, Lee TW, et al. Early results of endoscopic lung volume reduction for emphysema. J Thorac Cardiovasc Surg 2004;127(6):1564–73.

73. Strange C, Herth FJ, Kovitz KL, et al. VENT Study Group. Design of the Endobronchial Valve for Emphysema Palliation Trial (VENT): a non-surgical method of lung volume reduction. BMC Pulm Med 2007;7:10.

74. Brenner M, Hanna NM, Mina-Araghi R, et al. Innovative approaches to lung volume reduction for emphysema. Chest 2004;126(1):238–48.

75. Cardoso PF, Snell GI, Hopkins P, et al. Clinical application of airway bypass with paclitaxel-eluting stents: early results. J Thorac Cardiovasc Surg 2007;134(4):974–81.

76. Naunheim KS, Wood DE, Mohsenifar Z, et al. Long-term follow-up of patients receiving lung-volume-reduction surgery versus medical therapy for severe emphysema by the National Emphysema Treatment Trial Research Group. Ann Thorac Surg 2006;82(2): 431–43.

77. Fishman A, Martinez F, Naunheim K, et al. A randomized trial comparing lung-volume-reduction surgery with medical therapy for severe emphysema. N Engl J Med 2003;348(21):2059–73.

78. Goddard PR, Nicholson EM, Laszlo G, et al. Computed tomography in pulmonary emphysema. Clin Radiol 1982;33(4):379–87.

79. Choong CK, Macklem PT, Pierce JA, et al. Airway bypass improves the mechanical properties of explanted emphysematous lungs. Am J Respir Crit Care Med 2008;178(9):902–5.

80. Morrell NW, Wignall BK, Biggs T, et al. Collateral ventilation and gas exchange in emphysema. Am J Respir Crit Care Med 1994;150(3):635–41.

81. Abtin F, Goldin J, C Strange C, et al. The influence of fissural anatomy on the treatment outcome of patients with emphysema. Poster presentation at American Thoracic Society May, 2008, Toronto, Canada. Poster number 4036.

82. Abtin F, Goldin J, Brown M, et al. Variation in fissure anatomy in emphysema patients treated with endobronchial valve. Poster presentation at American Thoracic Society May, 2008, Toronto, Canada. Poster # 4125.

83. Ochs RA, Abtin F, Ghurabi R, et al. Computer-aided detection of endobronchial valves using volumetric CT. Acad Radiol 2009;16(2):172–80.

84. Newell JD, Hogg JC, Snider GL. Report of a workshop: quantitative computed tomography scanning in longitudinal studies of emphysema. Eur Respir J 2004;23:769–75.

85. Higuchi T, Reed A, Oto T, et al. Relation of interlobar collaterals to radiological heterogeneity in severe emphysema. Thorax 2006;61(5):409–13.

The National Emphysema Treatment Trial: Summary and Update

Melanie A. Edwards, MD[a],*, Stephen Hazelrigg, MD[b],
Keith S. Naunheim, MD[c]

KEYWORDS

- Lung volume reduction surgery • Surgery for emphysema
- The National Emphysema Treatment • Trial • Emphysema

In medicine one often encounters a disease process for which there is no clear path that will lead to the best outcome for all patients. Surgery for severe emphysema is one such problem. End stage emphysema patients are ravaged by progressive destruction of their lung parenchyma; they live with severe and progressive dyspnea, which results in a poor functional status and quality of life. Optimal medical therapy for severe emphysema includes smoking cessation, bronchodilators, antibiotics, steroids as indicated, and long-term domiciliary oxygen therapy, the only medical intervention that had been demonstrated to decrease mortality. It would thus seem that a surgical intervention that could lengthen survival, relieve dyspnea and improve both function and quality of life would be in high demand. Lung volume reduction (LVR) surgery was demonstrated to provide just such results in many clinical series in the 1990's and yet today is a rarely performed operation. The reason for this is difficult to pinpoint but lung volume reduction surgery (LVRS) has had a long and controversial history.

HISTORICAL BACKGROUND

Surgical therapy for severe emphysema developed with the primary objectives of palliating these patients by producing improvement in symptoms and quality of life. Previous operations tackled the problem of emphysema by the formation of pneumoperitoneum, phrenic nerve paralysis, thoracoplasty, lung denervation and tracheal stabilization and fixation with little sustained benefit and today these techniques remain of historical interest only.[1] The origins of lung volume reduction surgery stretch back to 1957 when Brantigan and Mueller first reported removing non-functional parts of the hyper-inflated lung parenchyma to improve dyspnea in emphysema patients.[2] Unfortunately, their procedure was not widely adopted in spite of a 75% reported clinical improvement. This was due to a relatively high mortality rate of 18% and the inability (due to technologic limitations) to provide objective evidence of a significant benefit.[2] Renewed interest in LVRS for the treatment of emphysema developed in the early 1990s after Wakabayashi published encouraging early results with unilateral thoracoscopic laser parenchymal ablation of giant bullous emphysema.[3] This garnered significant early enthusiasm and his updated analysis of 443 patients demonstrated an acceptable mortality rate of 4.8%, and 87% of patients reported symptomatic improvements.[4] These findings were not widely reproduced, and prospective data from Hazelrigg and colleagues showed only a modest 16% improvement in FEV_1 with laser ablation that did not

[a] Division of Thoracic Surgery, Louisiana State University, 1542 Tulane Avenue, Room 749, New Orleans, LA 70112, USA
[b] Division of Cardiothoracic Surgery, Department of Surgery, Southern Illinois University, Post Office Box 19638, Springfield, IL 62794-9638, USA
[c] Department of Cardiothoracic Surgery, St. Louis University Health Sciences Center, 3635 Vista Avenue at Grand, Post Office Box 15250, St. Louis, MO 63110-0250, USA
* Corresponding author.
E-mail address: edwmelanie@gmail.com (M.A. Edwards).

Thorac Surg Clin 19 (2009) 169–185
doi:10.1016/j.thorsurg.2009.02.007

favorably compare with contemporary results from stapled resections.[5] Joel Cooper's work helped to establish stapled resection as the procedure of choice for LVRS with his initial report of 20 patients in which he resected portions of both lungs via median sternotomy (MS). At a mean follow-up of 6.4 months, there were no deaths, and a significant 82% increase in FEV_1, with more moderate improvements in the distance walked in 6 minutes, dyspnea and quality of life scores, and a decline in the number of patients requiring supplemental oxygen therapy.[6] Even before the final publication of these findings, the fervor that was generated lead to the widespread adoption of LVRS at several centers. However, It is questionable whether the same careful patient selection and perioperative management was applied in all reported series as the resulting outcomes data yielded rather conflicting results. Although virtually all of these reports were favorable with morbidity and mortality ranging from 2.5%–10%,[7–13] a review of Medicare data from claims submitted between October 1995 and January 1996 showed much higher mortality rates of 14.4% and 23% at 3 and 12 months respectively. This report also documented very high rehospitalization rates and thus the Health Care Finance Administration (HCFA) decided to halt reimbursement for LVR unless and until definitive evidence was generated documenting efficacy.[14] This refusal to reimburse for LVR in the absence of a "definitive" study prompted the creation of the National Emphysema Treatment Trial (NETT), a multi-institutional study sponsored jointly by the National Heart, Lung and Blood Institute (NHLBI), and the Center for Medicare and Medicaid Services (CMS, formerly HCFA) to develop prospective randomized data on the outcomes of lung volume reduction surgery.[15]

NETT STUDY DESIGN

The National Emphysema Treatment Trial (NETT) was designed to compare short and long-term outcomes of best medical therapy for emphysema with best medical therapy plus LVRS. The primary questions were whether there was a sustained survival benefit with surgery and if such intervention improved lung function, exercise capacity and quality of life. The development of reproducible selection criteria for surgery was yet another important goal of the study. The NETT investigators chose survival and maximum exercise capacity measured by cycle ergometry as the primary outcome measures. Secondary measures of outcome included quality of life, both general and disease specific cost-effectiveness, pulmonary function and gas exchange, oxygen

requirement, 6 minute walk distance, cardiovascular measures and psychomotor functioning. Enrollment was limited to Medicare beneficiaries or those whose private insurance carrier would cover the costs of trial participation and CMS further stipulated that access to LVRS for Medicare patients could be obtained only through trial participation at one of the 17 designated clinical centers. The patient selection criteria included the presence of bilateral emphysema with severe airflow obstruction, hyperinflation on chest radiograph and the ability to participate in pulmonary rehabilitation. Eligible patients underwent comprehensive medical evaluation to exclude those who were at high risk for perioperative morbidity and mortality and those who had disease not suitable for LVRS or other circumstances that would make it unlikely for them to complete the trial. Clinical evaluations were performed at 6 and 12 months, then yearly thereafter.[15]

TREATMENT REGIMENS

Optimal medical therapy for emphysema was administered according to proposed guidelines from the American Thoracic Society and individual recommendations made by a NETT pulmonary physician. This included smoking cessation, bronchodilators, oxygen therapy, influenza and pneumococcal vaccinations, and pulmonary rehabilitation. All patients who were eligible for the study participated in pulmonary rehabilitation prerandomization for 6-10 weeks. The patients who had been randomized to medical therapy participated in intense pulmonary rehabilitation post-randomization for 8-9 weeks followed by long-term maintenance therapy over the trial duration.[15]

By consensus, bilateral stapled LVRS with excision of 20 to 35% of each lung was chosen as the surgical technique for the trial and the use of additional buttressing material was at the discretion of the individual surgeon. Bilateral LVRS had emerged as the standard of care in appropriate patients based on reports of operative morbidity/mortality rates similar to that of unilateral LVRS but with better technique improvement in pulmonary spirometric testing and patient-reported quality of life.[10,16] The surgical approach was by either median sternotomy or bilateral video-assisted thoracoscopic surgery (VATS), and in 6 centers, patients were randomized to either approach to try to identify any differences in outcome that may exist with the differing techniques. Patients randomized to the surgical arm of the study were expected to undergo operation within two weeks post randomization and resume pulmonary rehabilitation as soon as their clinical condition allowed.[15] Overall results from the NETT were first reported in 2003 after 2 years and in 2006, Naunheim and colleagues reported the long-term follow-up of the surviving LVRS patients at a median of 4.3 years.

SHORT TERM RESULTS

From January 1998 to December 2002, 3777 patients were evaluated at the 17 clinical centers, and 1218 were randomized after completing 6 to 10 weeks of pulmonary rehabilitation.[17] There were 608 patients assigned to surgery, and 610 to medical therapy. With the exception of a higher proportion of men in the medical therapy group, the base-line characteristics of both groups were similar (**Table 1**).[17]

All Patients

The primary outcome measures that the NETT intended to quantify were survival and change in exercise capacity. Exercise capacity was considered to be improved if there was a greater than 10 watt (W) increase above the post-rehabilitation baseline at the time of clinical evaluation. The median follow-up of patients was reported to be 29.2 months. Follow-up revealed a higher early mortality rate at 90 days in the surgery group (7.9%) as compared with the medical therapy group (1.3%), a result that was not unexpected considering the invasive nature of treatment in the surgical arm (**Table 2**).[17] There was no difference in the early mortality when one compared the VATS and median sternotomy approaches. Yet, despite the higher early mortality in the surgical group, there was no difference in overall mortality between the groups during the short-term follow-up (**Fig. 1**, panel A). There was, however, greater improvement experienced in functional status outcomes by patients in the surgical cohort when compared with their medical counterparts. This was evidenced by improvements in exercise capacity of more than 10 W in 28, 22 and 15% of LVR patients compared with improvements in only 4, 5 and 3% of medical patients after 6, 12 and 24 months (**Fig. 2**). When considering the secondary outcomes, the results also favored the group assigned to surgical therapy. They demonstrated a greater chance of having significant improvements in the 6 minute walk distance, percent of predicted FEV_1 and dyspnea. Additionally surgical patients noted greater improvement in general and health related quality of life, which had been defined as a decrease of more than 8 points on the St. George's Respiratory Questionnaire (SGRQ) (see **Fig. 2**; **Table 3**).[17]

High-Risk Subgroup

As the trial progressed, ongoing evaluation of the mortality data was performed by the data and safety monitoring board every 3 months. From these interim analyses, in April 2001, a high-risk patient subgroup emerged that demonstrated an increased risk of overall mortality after LVRS, characterized by a low FEV_1 and a homogenous pattern of emphysema.[18] Also associated with early increased mortality were a low FEV_1 and a low carbon monoxide diffusing capacity (DLCO) (**Fig. 3**). Based on the resulting information in May 2001 investigators ceased enrollment of patients with a low FEV_1 who had either a low carbon monoxide diffusing capacity, or homogenous emphysema on chest CT scan. All of the 140 patients in this group exhibited a very low FEV_1 of no more than 20%, and 87% of patients in this group had a carbon monoxide diffusing capacity of no more than 20% of their predicted value. On chest CT scanning, 94% of this group had a homogenous distribution of emphysema, and 41 patients met all three criteria. Among the 70 patients assigned to undergo surgery within this group, the overall mortality was 0.43 deaths per person-year versus 0.11 deaths per person-year in the 70 patients in medical arm.[18] No patients in the medical therapy group died at 30 days, in stark contrast to the 16% mortality rate at 30 days in the surgery group (**Table 4**). Updated analysis of this group was performed at 2 years and the poor outcomes with surgery continued to persist (see **Fig. 1**, panel B).[17] When analyzing the functional outcomes of the survivors from this subgroup at six months, the surgery group showed only small improvements in FEV_1, exercise capacity and the distance walked in 6 minutes. For these high-risk patients with low FEV_1 and either a low carbon monoxide diffusing capacity or homogenous emphysema, such small benefit was inconsequential given the prohibitive mortality risk and LVRS is not recommended for patients who meet these criteria.[18]

Non-High-Risk Patients

Exclusion of the patients in the high-risk subgroup left 1078 patients for analysis, and did not significantly alter the differences in mortality between the surgical group and the medical treatment group, although each group had a lower absolute mortality rate.[17] Patients assigned to LVRS continued to demonstrate higher short-term mortality, with 30-day rates of 2.2%, compared with 0.2% in the medical group, and 90-day mortality rates of 5.2% compared with 1.5% in

Table 1
Characteristics of all 1218 patients at baseline

Characteristic	Surgery Group (n = 608)	Medical-Therapy Group (n = 610)
Age at randomization – yr	66.5 ± 6.3	66.7 ± 5.9
Race or ethnic group – no. (%)	—	—
Non-Hispanic white	581 (96)	575 (94)
Non-Hispanic black	19 (3)	23 (4)
Other	8 (1)	12 (2)
Sex – no. (%)[†]	—	—
Female	253 (42)	219 (36)
Male	355 (58)	391 (64)
Distribution of emphysema on CT – no. (%)[a]	—	—
Predominantly upper lobe	385 (63)	405 (67)
Predominantly non-upper lobe	223 (37)	204 (33)
Heterogeneous	330 (54)	336 (55)
Homogeneous	278 (46)	274 (45)
Perfusion ratio[b]	0.30 ± 0.21	0.28 ± 0.23
Maximal workload – W	38.7 ± 21.1	39.4 ± 22.2
Distance walked in 6 min - ft[c]	1216.5 ± 312.6	1219.0 ± 316.0
FEV_1 after bronchodilator use - % of predicted value	26.8 ± 7.4	26.7 ± 7.0
Total lung capacity after bronchodilator use - % of predicted value	128.0 ± 15.3	128.5 ± 15.0
Residual volume after bronchodilator use - % of predicted value	220.5 ± 49.9	223.4 ± 48.9
Carbon monoxide diffusing capacity - % of predicted value	28.3 ± 9.7	28.4 ± 9.7
PaO_2 – mmHg	64.5 ± 10.5	64.2 ± 10.1
$PaCO_2$ – mmHg	43.3 ± 5.9	43.0 ± 5.8
Total score on St. George's Respiratory Questionnaire[d]	52.5 ± 12.6	53.6 ± 12.7
Average daily quality of well-being score**	0.58 ± 0.12	0.56 ± 0.11
Total UCSD shortness of breath score[e]	61.6 ± 18.1	63.4 ± 18.6

Baseline measurements were obtained after rehabilitation but before randomization, except for the carbon monoxide diffusing capacity, which was measured before rehabilitation. Plus-minus values are means ±SD. CT denotes computed tomography, FEV_1 forced expiratory volume in one second, PaO_2 partial pressure of arterial oxygen, and $PaCO_2$ partial pressure of arterial carbon dioxide.

[†] P for homogeneity = 0.04.

[a] Upper-lobe predominance of emphysema was judged subjectively by each center's radiologist, who described the distribution of disease as predominantly upper lobe, predominantly lower lobe, diffuse, or predominantly affecting superior segments of the lower lobes. The latter three choices were grouped as predominantly non-upper lobe. The classification of the emphysema as heterogeneous or homogeneous was based on subjective scores assigned by each center's radiologist to each of the three zones in each lung. Data on upper-lobe versus non-upper-lobe distribution were missing for one patient.

[b] The perfusion ratio is derived from the radionuclide perfusion scan. Each lung is divided into three zones, and a percentage of total perfusion is assigned to each zone. The ratio is calculated as the sum of the percentages assigned to the two upper zones divided by the sum of the percentages assigned to the four middle and lower zones.

[c] To convert values from feet to meters, divide by 3.28.

[d] The St. George's Respiratory Questionnaire is a 51-item questionnaire on the health-related quality of life with regard to respiratory symptoms that is completed by the patient; the total score ranges from 0 to 100, with lower scores indicating better health-related quality of life.

[e] The University of California. San Diego (UCSD), Shortness of Breath Questionnaire is a 24-item questionnaire about dyspnea that is completed by the patient; the total score ranges from 0 to 120, with lower scores indicating less shortness of breath.

the medical treatment arm (see **Table 2**). Early on, fewer surgical patients were living at home, as evidenced by a 28.1% rate of patients who were either hospitalized, living in a nursing facility or rehabilitation facility or unavailable for interview in spite of being alive. Such situations were observed in only 2.2% of patients in the medical group. Over the course of eight months, however,

Table 2
Mortality among all patients and in subgroups

Patients	90-Day Mortality			Total Mortality					
	Surgery Group	Medical-Therapy Group	P Value	Surgery Group		Medical-Therapy Group		Risk Ratio	P Value
	No. of Deaths/Total no. (% [95% CI])	No. of Deaths/Total no. (% [95% CI])		No. of Deaths/Total no.	No. of Deaths/Person-yr	No. of Deaths/Total no.	No. of Deaths/Person-yr		
All patients	48/608 (7.9 [5.9–10.3])	8/610 (1.3 [0.6–2.6])	<0.001	157/608	0.11	160/610	0.11	1.01	0.90
High-risk[a]	20/70 (28.6 [18.4–40.6])	0/70 (0 [0–5.1])	<0.001	42/70	0.33	30/70	0.18	1.82	0.06
Other	28/538 (5.2 [3.5–7.4])	8/540 (1.5 [0.6–2.9])	0.001	115/538	0.09	130/540	0.10	0.89	0.31
Subgroups[b]									
Patients with predominantly upper-lobe emphysema									
Low exercise capacity	4/139 (2.9 [0.8–7.2])	5/151 (3.3 [1.1–7.6])	1.00	26/139	0.07	51/151	0.15	0.47	0.005
High exercise capacity	6/206 (2.9 [1.1–6.2])	2/213 (0.9 [0.1–3.4])	0.17	34/206	0.07	39/213	0.07	0.98	0.70
Patients with predominantly non–upper-lobe emphysema									
Low exercise capacity	7/84 (8.3 [3.4–16.4])	0/65 (0 [0–5.5])	0.02	28/84	0.15	26/65	0.18	0.81	0.49
High exercise capacity	11/109 (10.1 [5.1–17.3])	1/111 (0.9 [0.02–4.9])	0.003	27/109	0.10	14/111	0.05	2.06	0.02

Mortality was measured from the date of randomization in both treatment groups. Total mortality rates are based on a mean follow-up of 29.2 months. P values were calculated by Fisher's exact test. Risk ratios are for the risk in the surgery group as compared with the risk in the medical-therapy group. A low base-line exercise capacity was defined as a post-rehabilitation base-line maximal workload at or below the sex-specific 40th percentile (25 W for women and 40 W for men); a high-exercise capacity was defined as a workload above this threshold. CI denotes confidence interval.

[a] High-risk patients were defined as those with a forced expiratory volume in one second (FEV₁) that was 20 percent or less of the predicted value and either homogeneous emphysema on computed tomography or a carbon monoxide diffusing capacity that was 20 percent or less of the predicted value.

[b] High-risk patients were excluded from the subgroup analyses. For total mortality, P for interaction = 0.004; this P value was derived from binary logistic-regression models with terms for treatment, subgroup, and the interaction between the two, with the use of an exact-score test with three degrees of freedom. Other factors that were considered as potential variables for the definition of subgroups included the base-line FEV_1, carbon monoxide diffusing capacity, partial pressure of arterial carbon dioxide, residual volume, ratio of residual volume to total lung capacity, ratio of expired ventilation in one minute to carbon dioxide excretion in one minute, distribution of emphysema (heterogeneous versus homogeneous), perfusion ratio, score for health-related quality of life, and Quality of Well-Being score; age; race or ethnic group; and sex.

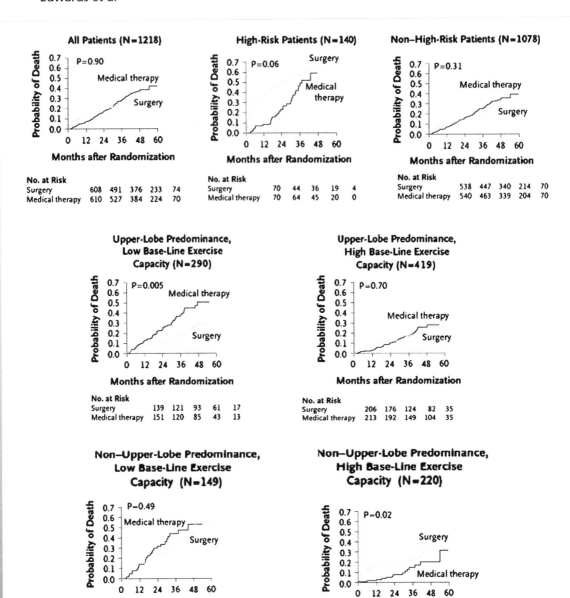

Fig. 1. The National Emphysema Treatment Trial (NETT): summary and update. Kaplan-Meier estimates of the probability of death as a function of the number of months after randomization. *P* values were derived by Fisher's exact test for the comparison between groups over a mean follow-up period of 29.2 months. High-risk patients were defined as those with a forced expiratory volume in one second that was 20 percent of less of the predicted value, and either homogeneous emphysema or a carbon monoxide diffusing capacity that was 20 percent of less of the predicted value. A low baseline exercise capacity was defined as a maximal workload at or below the sex-specific 40th percentile (25 W for women and 40 W for men); a high exercise capacity was defined as a workload above this threshold. This was an intention-to-treat analysis. (*From* Fishman A, Martinez F, Naunheim K, et al. A randomized trial comparing lung-volume-reduction surgery with medical therapy for severe emphysema. N Engl J Med 2003;348:2059–73; with permission. Copyright © 2003, Massachusetts Medical Society.)

this difference dissipated such that 3.3% of the surgical patients and 3.7% of medical patients were institutionalized, a difference that was not significant.[17]

Also, over time the observed mortality differences ceased to be significant. In the non-high-risk group of patients, the total mortality rates of 0.09 deaths per person-year in the surgery group,

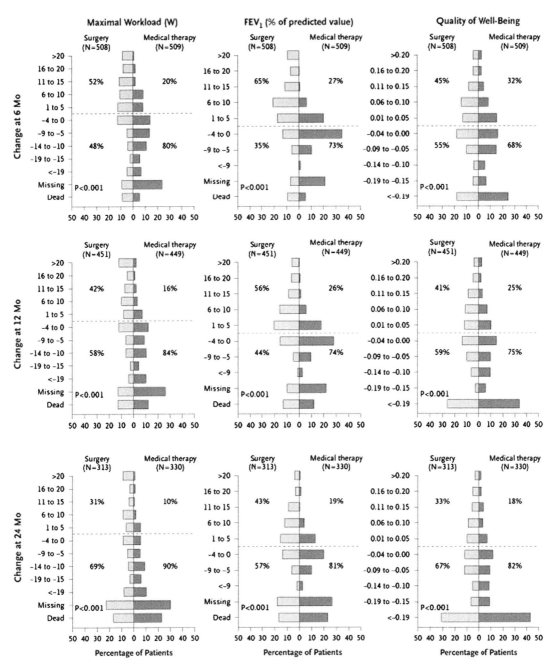

Fig. 2. Histograms of changes from baseline in exercise capacity (maximal workload), percentage of the predicted value for forced expiratory volume in one second (FEV₁), and quality of life (quality of well-being score) after 6, 12, and 24 months of follow-up. Baseline measurements were performed after pulmonary rehabilitation. Patients previously identified as high-risk were excluded. Patients who were too ill to complete the procedure or who declined to complete the procedure but did not explain why were included in the "missing" category. For the quality of well-being score, patients who died were assigned a score of 0 on the questionnaire for the visit. *P* values were determined by the Wilcoxon rank-sum test. The degree to which the bars are shifted to the upper left of the chart indicates the degree of relative benefit of lung-volume-reduction surgery over medical treatment. The percentage shown in each quadrant is the percentage of patients in the specified treatment group with a change in the outcome falling into that quadrant. This was an intention-to-treat analysis. (*From* Fishman A, Martinez F, Naunheim K, et al. A randomized trial comparing lung-volume-reduction surgery with medical therapy for severe emphysema. N Engl J Med 2003;348:2059–73; with permission. Copyright © 2003, Massachusetts Medical Society.)

Table 3
Improvement in exercise capacity and health-related quality of life at 24 months

Patients	Improvement in Exercise Capacity				Improvement in Health-Related Quality of Life			
	Surgery Group	Medical-Therapy Group	Odds Ratio	P Value	Surgery Group	Medical-Therapy Group	Odds Ratio	P Value
	no./total no. (%)	—		no./total no. (%)	—	—		—
All patients	54/371 (15)	10/378 (3)	6.27	<0.001	121/371 (33)	34/378 (9)	4.90	<0.001
High-risk[a]	4/58 (7)	1/48 (2)	3.48	0.37	6/58 (10)	0/48	—	0.03
Other	50/313 (16)	9/330 (3)	6.78	<0.001	115/313 (37)	34/330 (10)	5.06	<0.001
Subgroups[b]								
Predominantly upper-lobe emphysema			—			—		
Low exercise capacity	25/84 (30)	0/92	—	<0.001	40/84 (48)	9/92 (10)	8.38	<0.001
High exercise capacity	17/115 (15)	4/138 (3)	5.81	0.001	47/115 (41)	15/138 (11)	5.67	<0.001
Predominantly non-upper-lobe emphysema								
Low exercise capacity	6/49 (12)	3/41 (7)	1.77	0.50	18/49 (37)	3/41 (7)	7.35	0.001
High exercise capacity	2/65 (3)	2/59 (3)	0.90	1.00	10/65 (15)	7/59 (12)	1.35	0.61

Improvement in exercise capacity in patients followed for 24 months after randomization was defined as an increase in the maximal workload of more than 10 W from the patient's post-rehabilitation base-line value. Improvement in the health-related quality of life in patients followed for 24 months after randomization was defined as a decrease in the score on the St. George's Respiratory Questionnaire of more than 8 points (on a 100-point scale) from the patient's post-rehabilitation base-line score. For both analyses, patients who died or who missed the 24-month assessment were considered not to have improvement. Odds ratios are for improvement in the surgery group as compared with the medical therapy group. P values were calculated by Fisher's exact test. A low base-line exercise capacity was defined as a post-rehabilitation base-line maximal workload at or below the sex-specific 40th percentile (25 W for women and 40 W for men); a high exercise capacity was defined as a workload above this threshold.

[a] High-risk patients were excluded from the subgroup analyses. For improvement in exercise capacity, P for interaction = 0.005; for improvement in health-related quality of life, P for interaction = 0.03. These P values were derived from binary logistic-regression models with terms for treatment, subgroup, and the interaction between the two, with the use of an exact-score test with three degrees of freedom. Other factors that were considered as potential variables for the definition of subgroups included the base-line FEV$_1$, carbon monoxide diffusing capacity, partial pressure of arterial carbon dioxide, residual volume, ratio of residual volume to total lung capacity, ratio of expired ventilation in one minute to carbon dioxide excretion in one minute, distribution of emphysema (heterogeneous versus. homogeneous), perfusion ratio, score for health related quality of life, and Quality of Well-Being score; age; race or ethnic group; and sex.

[b] High-risk patients were defined as those with a forced expiratory volume in one second (FEV1) that was 20 percent or less of the predicted value and either homogeneous emphysema on computed tomography or a carbon monoxide diffusing capacity that was 20 percent or less of the predicted value.

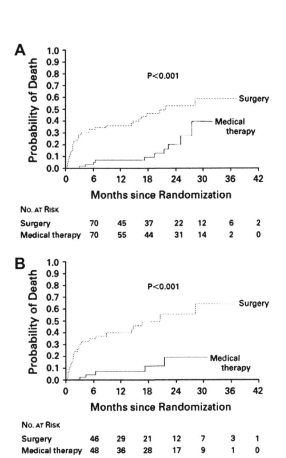

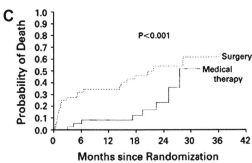

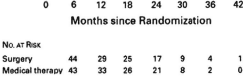

Fig. 3. Kaplan-Meier estimates of the probability of death among high-risk patients, according to whether they were randomly assigned to undergo lung-volume-reduction surgery or receive medical therapy. This intention-to-treat analysis shows the overall results for the high-risk group (*A*), the subgroup of patients with an FEV_1 that was no more than 20 percent of their predicted value and a homogeneous distribution of emphysema on CT scanning (*B*), and the subgroup of patients with an FEV_1 that was no more than 20 percent of their predicted value (*C*). For each analysis the difference between groups was significant (*P*<.001, *P*<.001, and *P* = .005, respectively) by the log-rank test. (*From* The National Emphysema Treatment Trial Research Group. Patients at high risk of death after lung-volume-reduction surgery. N Engl J Med 2001;345:1075–83; with permission. Copyright © 2001, Massachusetts Medical Society.)

and 0.10 deaths per person-year in the medical therapy group were not significantly different at 29 months (see **Fig. 1**, panel C). As similarly demonstrated in the overall analysis, there were more favorable results with surgery with respect to the changes in exercise capacity, distance walked in 6 minutes, percent predicted FEV_1, quality of life and degree of dyspnea at 6, 12 and 24 months (see **Fig. 2**; **Table 3**).[17] Patients who were not designated as being at high risk for mortality could reasonably expect some functional gains and improvements in health-related quality of life in the short term, however they did not gain a significant survival benefit.

Preoperative Predictors of Outcome Among Non-High-Risk Patients

Throughout the trial, investigators and the data and safety monitoring board analyzed groups of patients who may possibly derive so much benefit from the procedure as to mandate their removal from the trial. No such group emerged, and in the short-term the only preoperative factors predictive of mortality that gained significance were the presence or absence of upper-lobe predominant emphysema on chest CT, and the level of baseline exercise capacity.[17] The cutoff point for defining low baseline exercise capacity that predicted the differential risk of death was the 40th percentile, 25 W for women, and 40 W for men. Only the distribution of emphysema could be related to improvements in the maximal achievable workload at 24 months and none of the multiple baseline factors examined predicted improvements in health related quality of life. Thus, using these 2 characteristics (emphysema distribution and exercise capacity), patients were subdivided into 4 groups to further characterize the risks and benefits from LVRS, producing strong evidence of differential effects of these groupings on the risk of death, and changes in exercise capacity at 24 months.[17]

Upper-Lobe Disease and Low Baseline Exercise Capacity

There were a total of 290 patients identified who had both upper-lobe disease and low baseline exercise capacity. Patients in this sub-group who underwent LVRS had a significant survival advantage in the short-term with 0.47 risk ratio of death (see **Fig. 1**, panel D), and 30% of these surgical patients demonstrated improvements in the maximum workload relative to 0% of medical therapy patients, a difference that was significant. Surgical patients were also more likely than medically treated patients to have an 8-point

Table 4
Mortality rates among high-risk patients

Variable	30-Day Mortality[a]				Overall Mortality[b]				Risk Ratio (95% CI) for Surgery Versus Medical Therapy
	Surgery		Medical Therapy		Surgery		Medical Therapy		
	No. of patients	No. of deaths (% [95% CI])	No. of patients	No. of deaths	No. of deaths/ total no. of patients	Death rate/ patient-yr	No. of deaths/ total no. of patients	Death rate/ patient-yr	
High-risk group overall	69[c]	11 (16 [8.2–26.7])	70	0	33/70	0.43	10/70	0.11	3.94 (1.9–9.0)
Subgroup									
FEV₁ «20% of predicted and homogeneous emphysema	45[c]	8 (18 [8.0–32.1])	48	0[c]	23/46	0.50	5/48	0.08	5.96 (2.2–20.1)
FEV₁ «20% of predicted and DLCO «20% of predicted	44	8 (18 [8.2–32.7])	43	0[d]	22/44	0.42	8/43	0.14	2.98 (1.3–7.7)

High-risk patients are those with a forced expiratory volume in one second (FEV₁) that was no more than 20 percent of their predicted value and either a homogeneous distribution of emphysema on CT scanning or a carbon monoxide diffusing capacity (DLCO) that was no more than 20 percent of their predicted value. A total of 41 patients had all three risk factors (FEV₁ «20 percent of the predicted value, a homogeneous distribution of emphysema on CT scanning, and a DLCO «20 percent of the predicted value): 20 in the surgery group and 21 in the medical-therapy group. Five of the 20 patients in the surgery group who had all three factors died within 30 days after surgery. CI denotes confidence interval.

P<.001 for the comparison with the surgery group.

P = .002 for the comparison with the surgery group.

[a] The 30-day mortality rate was measured from the date of surgery for those in the surgery group and from the date of randomization for those in the medical-therapy group.

[b] The analysis was conducted according to the intention to treat. The overall mortality rate was measured from the date of randomization.

[c] One patient in the high-risk subgroup who was assigned to surgery declined to undergo it and was excluded from this analysis.

[d] P = .006 for the comparison with the surgery group.

improvement in the SGRQ score at 24 months (48% versus 10%) (see **Table 3**).[17]

Upper-Lobe Disease and High Baseline Exercise Capacity

For the 419 patients with upper-lobe disease and high exercise capacity, LVRS did not show any survival advantages when compared with medical therapy (see **Fig. 1**, panel E).[13] However, more of these patients improved greater than 10 W in the maximal workload achieved, and a higher proportion also had quality of life improvement with a greater than eight-point decrease in the SGRQ at 24 months (see **Table 3**).[17]

Non-Upper-Lobe Disease and Low Baseline Exercise Capacity

Within the group of 149 patients with non-upper-lobe disease and low exercise capacity there was no difference in the risk of death between the surgical and medical therapy groups (see **Fig. 1**, panel F), nor were there significant relative improvements in exercise capacity. There was, however, significant improvement in health related quality of life in the LVRS patients observed at 24 months (37% versus 7%) (see **Table 3**).[17]

Non-Upper Lobe Disease and High Baseline Exercise Capacity

Patients who had non-upper lobe predominant disease and high exercise capacity and underwent LVRS had a higher risk of death than those in the medical therapy group, with a risk ratio of 2.06 (see **Fig. 1**, panel G and **Table 2**).[17] Additionally, the likelihood of improvement in the maximal workload and health related quality of life scores were similarly low in both the surgical and medical therapy groups at 3% each (see **Table 3**).[17] In spite of the unfavorable results in this group of patients, identifying and defining their characteristics was one of the important secondary goals of the trial.

Thus, when considering the NETT primary outcome measures of survival and changes in exercise capacity, the most convincing advantages of LVRS over medical therapy were found in those patients who had both upper-lobe predominant disease and low baseline exercise capacity. There was clearly no benefit from surgery in patients with non-upper-lobe disease and high exercise capacity, a subgroup that demonstrated a higher risk of death. In the remaining two subgroups, although there was no difference in survival between LVRS and medical therapy, there were differences in functional outcomes. Lung volume reduction surgery produced improvements in both baseline exercise capacity and health related quality of life in the subgroup with upper-lobe predominant disease and high exercise capacity. The non-upper-lobe predominant disease and low exercise capacity subgroup experienced no exercise improvement with LVRS, but did demonstrate a benefit in health-related quality of life at 24 months.[17]

OPERATIVE MORBIDITY AND MORTALITY

A more focused analysis of the morbidity and mortality data from the NETT was undertaken by Naunheim and colleagues, as they examined the 511 non-high-risk patients who underwent LVRS, with the intent of identifying predictors of operative mortality, and pulmonary and cardiovascular morbidity. Due to the fragile nature of patients with severe emphysema it was important to understand the "clinical cost" at which the benefits derived from LVRS were obtained. The 90-day mortality from all causes was chosen to represent the most accurate risk of mortality as many of these patients had prolonged stays in acute care hospitals and chronic care facilities. They found an operative mortality of 5.5% in this non-high risk surgical cohort, and an incidence of major pulmonary and cardiac morbidity of 29.8% and 20% respectively. As suggested in the NETT subgroup analysis, the only significant prognostic factor for operative mortality was the presence of non-upper-lobe predominant disease on chest CT as characterized by a radiologist. Major pulmonary morbidity was predicted by age, percent-predicted FEV_1, and percent-predicted DLCO. Patients with advanced age, oral steroid use and non-upper-lobe predominant disease by quantitative image analysis were found to be at higher risk for cardiovascular complications.[19] The relatively low mortality rates demonstrated in the NETT trial spoke to the critical importance of careful patient selection, preoperative optimization of functional status and attention to perioperative care when selecting and managing patients undergoing LVRS.

Median Sternortomy Versus Vats

The development of contemporary surgical therapy for severe emphysema began with Joel Cooper 's revival of lung volume reduction surgery in 1994. Unlike Brantigan in the 1950s, Cooper approached his bilateral pulmonary resections by median sternotomy.[3] The concurrent development and increasing application of video-assisted thoracoscopic surgery (VATS) during this same time period made it a viable alternative approach to median sternotomy in the performance of LVR procedure. While evidence mounted regarding the benefit of a bilateral over a unilateral LVRS,[10,16] the optimal operative approach had not been similarly elucidated. A secondary goal of the NETT was to examine and compare the outcomes of median sternotomy compared with VATS for mortality, morbidity and functional outcome. Across the NETT centers, 6 sites performed both median sternotomy and VATS and their patients were randomized to either technique. In the remaining 11 centers VATS LVR only was performed at 3, and median sternotomy only at 8. In the randomized patient subset, there were no intraoperative deaths in either group, and the 30 and 90-day mortality rates were similar. When considering the entire surgical cohort (randomized and otherwise) there were no significant differences with regards to complications or functional outcomes. The only difference noted was that the use of median sternotomy was associated with a longer length of stay and higher operative costs at 6 months when compared with VATS. This difference that was maintained across non-randomized and randomized comparison groups.[20]

LONG-TERM OUTCOMES

Would the benefits derived from surgery last? Important concerns regarding the durability of the survival benefits, and improvements in functional status were addressed as the NETT investigators continued to monitor patients after the completion of the initial trial. There are four subgroups of patients defined by the presence or absence of upper-lobe predominant disease in combination with baseline exercise capacity (high or low).

All Patients

Seventy percent of surviving patients participated in the extension of follow up, and 76% participated in the mailed quality of life data collection. At a median follow-up period of 4.3 years, 283 patients assigned to LVRS and 324 assigned to medical therapy had died. From this data, a significant survival advantage eventually emerged in the entire surgical group with 0.11 deaths per person-year compared with the medical group in which there were 0.13 deaths per person-year (**Fig. 4**, panel A).[21] In addition to the survival benefit, improvements in exercise capacity of more than 10 W above the post-rehabilitation baseline were seen in a significantly higher number of surgical patients relative to medical patients at all time points up to 3 years, with improvements seen in 23%, 15% and 9% of LVRS patients, compared with 5%, 3% and 1% of medical patients at 1, 2

and 3 years (**Fig. 5**, panel A). Similarly, improvements in health-related quality of life were significantly better in the surgical group up to 5 years with 40%, 32%, 20%, 10% and 13% of LVRS patients demonstrating a greater than 8-point decrease in the SGRQ, versus 9%, 8%, 8%, 4% and 7% improvements in the medical group at 1, 2, 3, 4, and 5 years (**Fig. 6**, panel A).[21]

High-Risk Patients

As seen in the 2-year follow-up, the high-risk subgroup continued to demonstrate a substantial mortality risk from LVRS with no derived functional benefit.

Non-High Risk Patients

Updated analysis of the 1078 non-high-risk patients also revealed a significant survival advantage for LVRS, with mortality rates of 0.10 deaths per person-year in the LVRS group, and 0.12 deaths per person-year in the medical group (see **Fig. 4**, panel B). Although exercise capacity improved with LVRS and the benefit over medical therapy was sustained, patients in both medical and surgical groups experienced gradual declines over a 3-year period (see **Fig. 5**, panel B). Measures of health related quality of life were also better for LVRS patients in this updated analysis with sustained, significant improvements in SGRQ in 43%, 35%, 22%, 12% and 15% of LVRS patients at 1, 2, 3, 4, and 5 years respectively, while only 10%, 9%, 8%, 5% and 7% of medical patients derived any benefit over the same time period (see **Fig. 6**, panel B).[21]

Upper-Lobe Emphysema with Low Exercise Capacity

In the 290 patients with upper-lobe disease and low exercise capacity, a survival advantage for LVRS was maintained throughout the 5 years of follow up (see **Fig. 4**, panel C). Lung volume reduction surgery patients also continued to demonstrate more significant improvements in exercise capacity (see **Fig. 5**, panel C) and SGRQ score with surgical therapy over the same time period.

Upper Lobe and High Exercise Capacity

The cohort of 419 patients with upper-lobe emphysema and high exercise capacity continued to see no survival benefit from LVRS, however they still enjoyed better functional outcomes as evidenced by a significantly greater proportion of patients who had improved exercise capacity (see **Fig. 5**, panel D) and SGRQ scores (see **Fig. 6**, panel D) with surgery.

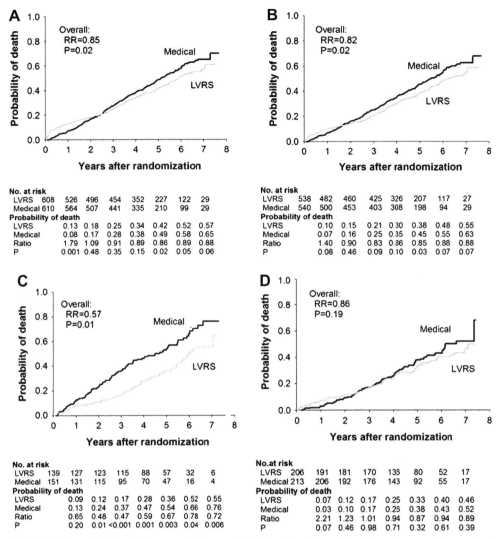

Fig. 4. Kaplan-Meier estimates of the cumulative probability of death as a function of years after randomization to lung volume reduction surgery (*LVRS, gray line*) or medical treatment (*black line*) for (*A*) all patients and (*B–D*) non-high-risk and upper-lobe-predominant subgroups of patients. The *P* value is from the Fisher exact test for difference in the proportions of patients who died during the 4.3 years (median) of follow-up. Shown below each graph are the numbers of patients at risk, the Kaplan-Meier probabilities, the ratio of the probabilities (LVRS:Medical), and *P* value for the difference in these probabilities. This is an intention-to-treat analysis. (*A*) All patients (N = 1218). (*B*) Non-high-risk patients (n = 1078). (*C*) Upper-lobe-predominant and low baseline exercise capacity (n = 290). (*D*) Upper-lobe-predominant and high exercise capacity (n = 419). (RR = relative risk.) (*From* Naunheim KS, Wood DE, Mohsenifar Z, et al. Long-term follow-up of patients receiving lung-volume-reduction surgery versus medical therapy for severe emphysema by the National Emphysema Treatment Trial research group. Ann Thorac Surg 2006;82:431–43; with permission.)

Non-Upper Lobe with High Exercise Capacity

Initially these patients were found to only have significant improvements in health-related quality of life with LVRS compared with medical therapy at two years with no benefit in either survival or exercise capacity. Unfortunately, even this modest benefit disappeared by 3 years, leaving no advantage to LVRS for these patients.

Non-Upper Lobe with Low Exercise Capacity

These patients who at two years failed to demonstrate any benefit from LVRS were found not to gain any benefit long term from the LVRS procedure with regard to survival, quality of life, or exercise capacity.[21]

Although there were declines in most of the absolute outcome measures in both treatment

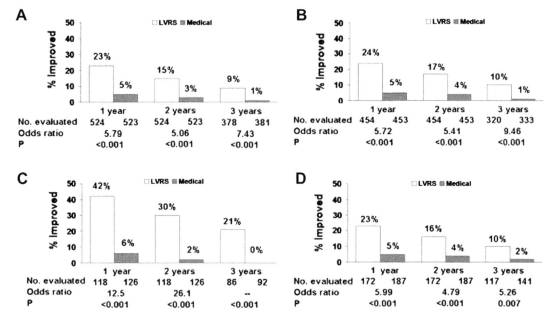

Fig. 5. Improvement in exercise capacity (increase in maximum work of >10 W above the patient's postrehabilitation baseline) at 1, 2, and 3 years after randomization to lung volume reduction surgery (*LVRS, open box*) or medical treatment (*filled box*) for (*A*) all patients and (*B–D*) non-high-risk and upper-lobe-predominant subgroups of patients. Shown below each graph are the numbers of patients evaluated, the odds ratio for improvement (LVRS:Medical), and the Fisher exact *P* value for difference in proportion improved. Patients who died or who did not complete the assessment were considered not improved. This is an intention-to-treat analysis. (*A*) All patients (N = 1218). (*B*) Non-high-risk patients (n = 1078). (*C*) Upper-lobe-predominant and low baseline exercise capacity (n = 290). (*D*) Upper-lobe-predominant and high exercise capacity (n = 419). (*From* Naunheim KS, Wood DE, Mohsenifar Z, et al. Long-term follow-up of patients receiving lung-volume-reduction surgery versus medical therapy for severe emphysema by the National Emphysema Treatment Trial research group. Ann Thorac Surg 2006;82:431–43; with permission.)

groups over time, LVRS patients were significantly better off than their medical counterparts at each time period with regard to exercise capacity and health related quality of life.

COST EFFECTIVENESS

During the development and enrollment phases of the NETT, emphysema was estimated to affect approximately 2 million Americans,[22] and more recent estimates suggest that the incidence has essentially doubled to approximately 4 million Americans.[23] Given the chronic, debilitating nature of emphysema, and its growing prevalence, the economic impact of treating these patients, either with surgical or medical therapy, has the potential to be quite significant. New therapies need to be evaluated within this context, in addition to examining the more traditional outcome measures such as survival, functional gains and quality of life estimates. As such, within the NETT, separate, concurrent prospective analysis of the cost-effectiveness of LVRS was conducted to quantify the actual economic impact of LVRS using costs per

quality-adjusted life years gained.[24] At both the short, and long-term follow-up, LVRS was found to be costly relative to medical therapy, even when the high-risk subgroup had been excluded.[25,26] However, at long-term follow-up the cost-effectiveness of LVRS was more favorable, especially when compared with standard surgical therapies for other conditions. In spite of this, the fact remains that LVRS is still perceived by many as carrying a prohibitive expense. This is possibly one of the reasons that, in spite of CMS approval for LVRS, the procedure has not experienced widespread acceptance and application.

PULMONARY REHABILITATION

Pulmonary rehabilitation was an integral part of the care of the patients in the NETT, and whenever possible, patients were enrolled in rehabilitation at one of the primary NETT centers, however, a significant proportion (65%) were treated at satellite centers with programs that were developed and supervised by the NETT center.[27] There were

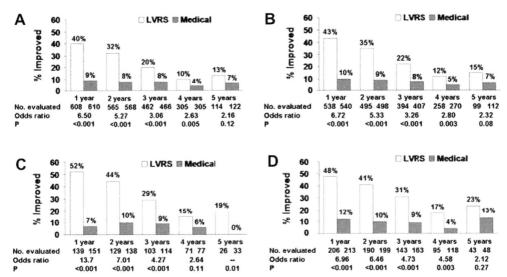

Fig. 6. Improvement in health-related quality of life (decrease in St. George 's Respiratory Questionnaire total score of >8 units below the patient 's postrehabilitation baseline) at 1, 2, 3, 4, and 5 years after randomization to lung volume reduction surgery (*LVRS, open box*) or medical treatment (*filled box*) for (*A*) all patients and (*B–D*) non-high-risk and upper-lobe-predominant subgroups of patients. Shown below each graph are the numbers of patients evaluated, the odds ratio for improvement (LVRS:Medical), and the Fisher exact *P* value for difference in proportion improved. Patients who died or who did not complete the assessment were considered not improved. This is an intention-to-treat analysis. (*A*) All patients (n = 1218). (*B*) Non-high-risk patients (n = 1078). (*C*) Upper-lobe-predominant and low baseline exercise capacity (n = 290). (*D*) Upper-lobe-predominant and high exercise capacity (n = 419). (*From* Naunheim KS, Wood DE, Mohsenifar Z, et al. Long-term follow-up of patients receiving lung-volume-reduction surgery versus medical therapy for severe emphysema by the National Emphysema Treatment Trial research group. Ann Thorac Surg 2006;82:431–43; with permission.)

some patients who could not complete the course of rehabilitation therapy and thus proved too debilitated to undergo randomization. Conversely, a number of participants derived sufficient benefits that they were unwilling to undergo surgery and were also excluded from randomization. Of interest, although some patients experienced significant improvements in most measures of exercise capacity, dyspnea and quality of life after pulmonary rehabilitation, these changes did not translate into improved outcomes with surgery. Instead the subgroup with low exercise capacity achieved greater gains in functional status and survival benefit with LVRS indicating that patients who do not significantly improve after pulmonary rehabilitation may be more likely to benefit from LVRS. Overall, the NETT provided important validation of the role of pulmonary rehabilitation in preoperative evaluation and preparation for LVRS and also demonstrated that these results could be obtained at in the general community.[27,28]

SUMMARY

Surgery for severe emphysema involves a cohort of patients who are already at risk for increased perioperative morbidity and mortality. Through the careful screening and selection process, improved intraoperative techniques and rigorous attention to postoperative care, the NETT managed to yield acceptable improvements in survival and functional outcomes in this fragile patient cohort and these benefits were sustained over the long-term. Identification of the characteristics associated with a higher risk of death has provided tangible patient selection criteria for the ongoing application of LVRS. Because the NETT was such a large-scale study, the protocols that were developed had to be standardized across several centers. This produced reliable and reproducible standards for evaluation and treatment that can be applied to the surgical treatment of emphysema.

When considering these criteria, although individualized patient selection is important, only patients with upper-lobe predominant disease on chest CT and possibly those with non-upper-lobe predominant disease who also have low baseline exercise capacity are appropriate candidates for LVRS. Expectedly, questions remain regarding the exact mechanism whereby the benefits derived from LVRS are obtained. Additionally, the benefit of LVRS in patients with heterogeneous but non-upper-lobe predominant disease remains to be further elucidated.

In spite of the limitations of the study, the NETT, through a tremendous coordinated effort, provided valuable outcomes data, answered the pressing questions regarding lung volume reduction surgery that existed at the time, and provided valuable insight into other facets of emphysema physiology and management through direct observation.

Based on the NETT findings, in November 2003, CMS published criteria for expanded coverage for LVRS to include non-high-risk patients who demonstrated either upper-lobe predominant emphysema, or non-upper-lobe predominant emphysema and low baseline exercise capacity and who met the screening guidelines.[29] This study not only provided data regarding the clinical efficacy of LRVS, but it was instrumental in determining health policy guidelines for the surgical management of emphysema.

REFERENCES

1. Deslauriers J. History of surgery for emphysema. Semin Thorac Cardiovasc Surg 1996;8:43–51.
2. Brantigan OC, Mueller E. Surgical treatment of pulmonary emphysema. Am Surg 1957;23:789–804.
3. Wakabayashi A, Brenner M, Kayaleh RA, et al. Thoracoscopic carbon dioxide laser treatment of bullous emphysema. Lancet 1991;337:881–3.
4. Wakabayashi A. Thoracoscopic laser pneumoplasty in the treatment of diffuse bullous emphysema. Ann Thorac Surg 1995;60:936–42.
5. Hazelrigg S, Boley T, Henkle J, et al. Thoracoscopic laser bullectomy: a prospective study with three-month results. J Thorac Cardiovasc Surg 1996;112:319–26.
6. Cooper JD, Trulock EP, Triantafillou AN, et al. Bilateral pneumectomy (volume reduction) for chronic obstructive pulmonary disease. J Thorac Cardiovasc Surg 1995;109:106–16.
7. Cooper JD, Patterson GA, Sundaresan RS, et al. Results of 150 consecutive bilateral lung volume reduction procedures in patients with severe emphysema. J Thorac Cardiovasc Surg 1996;112:1319–30.
8. Bingisser R, Zollinger A, Hauser M, et al. Bilateral volume reduction surgery for diffuse pulmonary emphysema by video-assisted thoracoscopy. J Thorac Cardiovasc Surg 1996;112:875–82.
9. Miller JI Jr, Lee RB, Mansour KA. Lung volume reduction surgery: lessons learned. Ann Thorac Surg 1996;61:1464–9.
10. McKenna RJ Jr, Brenner M, Fischel RJ, et al. Should lung volume reduction surgery be unilateral or bilateral? J Thorac Cardiovasc Surg 1996;112:1331–9.
11. Daniel TM, Chan BK, Bhaskar V, et al. Lung volume reduction surgery. Case selection, operative technique, and clinical results. Ann Surg 1996;223:526–33.
12. Argenziano M, Moazami N, Thomashow B, et al. Extended indications for volume reduction pneumoplasty in advanced emphysema. Ann Thorac Cardiovasc Surg 1996;62:1588–97.
13. Wisser W, Tschernko E, Senbaklavaci O, et al. Functional improvement after volume reduction: sternotomy versus videoendoscopic approach. Ann Thorac Surg 1997;63:822–8.
14. Heath Care Financing Administration. Report to congress. Lung volume reduction surgery and Medicare coverage policy: implications of recently published evidence. Baltimore (MD): Heath Care Financing Administration; 1998.
15. National Emphysema Treatment Trial Research Group. Rationale and design of the National Emphysema Treatment Trial (NETT): a prospective randomized trial of lung volume reduction surgery. J Thorac Cardiovasc Surg 1999;118:518–28.
16. Lowdermilk GA, Keenan RJ, Landreneau RJ, et al. Comparison of clinical results for unilateral and bilateral thoracoscopic lung volume reduction. Ann Thorac Surg 2000;69:1670–4.
17. National Emphysema Treatment Trial Research Group. A randomized trial comparing lung-volume-reduction surgery with medical therapy for severe emphysema. N Engl J Med 2003;348:2059–73.
18. National Emphysema Treatment Trial Research Group. Patients at high risk of death after lung-volume-reduction surgery. N Engl J Med 2001;345:1075–83.
19. Naunheim KS, Wood DE, Krasna MJ, et al. Predictors of operative mortality and cardiopulmonary morbidity in the National Emphysema Treatment Trial. J Thorac Cardiovasc Surg 2006;131:43–53.
20. National Emphysema Treatment Trial Research Group. Safety and efficacy of median sternotomy versus video-assisted thoracic surgery for lung volume reduction surgery. J Thorac Cardiovasc Surg 2004;127:1350–60.
21. Naunheim KS, Wood DE, Mohsenifar Z, et al. Long-term follow-up of patients receiving lung-volume-reduction surgery versus medical therapy for severe emphysema by the National Emphysema Treatment Trial research group. Ann Thorac Surg 2006;82:431–43.
22. National Center for Health Statistics. National Health Interview Survey 1994. Available at: http://www.cdc.gov/nchs/data/series/sr_10/sr10_193acc.pdf. Accessed May 9, 2008.
23. National Center for Health Statistics. National Health Interview Survey 2006. Available at: http://www.cdc.gov/nchs/data/series/sr_10/sr10_235.pdf. Accessed May 9, 2008.
24. Ramsey SD, Sullivan SD, Kaplan RM, et al. Economic analysis of lung volume reduction surgery as part of the National Emphysema Treatment Trial. Ann Thorac Surg 2001;71:995–1002.
25. National Emphysema Treatment Trial Research Group. Cost effectiveness of lung-volume-reduction

surgery for patients with severe emphysema. N Engl J Med 2003;348:2092–102.

26. Ramsey SD, Shroyer AL, Sullivan SD, et al. Updated evaluation of the cost-effectiveness of lung volume reduction surgery. Chest 2007;131:823–32.

27. Ries AL, Make BJ, Lee SM, et al. The effects of pulmonary rehabilitation in the National Emphysema Treatment Trial. Chest 2005;128:3799–809.

28. Ries AL, Make BJ, Reilly JJ. Pulmonary rehabilitation in emphysema. Proc Am Thorac Soc 2008;5: 524–9.

29. Centers for Medicare and Medicaid Services. Revision 240.1 of pub. 100–03 Medicare national coverage determinations. Available at: http://www.cms.hhs.gov/transmittals/downloads/R3NCD.pdf. Accessed May 17, 2008.

Staged Lung Volume Reduction Surgery—Rationale and Experience

David Waller, MD, FRCS (CTh), FCCP*, Inger Oey, MD, FRCS

KEYWORDS

- COPD • Emphysema • Video-assisted thoracoscopy
- Lung volume reduction surgery • Health status

Lung volume reduction surgery (LVRS) relieves the sensation of breathlessness by reducing the hyperinflation of the thoracic cavity associated with air trapping in emphysema.[1] The conventional approach to LVRS has been to remove lung tissue bilaterally at one operation to achieve the operative goal.[2] If, however, one assumes that the thoracic cavity is not composed of two fixed compartments and that the mediastinum is free to move, then removing lung tissue from one hemithorax will relieve the effects of hyperinflation on both sides. The authors previously produced supportive evidence that unilateral LVRS results in physiological and health status improvements.[3]

By virtue of the poor condition of those who need LVRS, it is a high-risk procedure. There is evidence that a unilateral approach may reduce postoperative morbidity and mortality.[4] This is particularly so if lung volume reduction can be achieved by video- assisted thoracoscopic surgery (VATS) rather than median sternotomy,[5] which is likely to result in a shorter hospital stay and faster recovery.[3] The authors advocate VATS as the method of choice for LVRS in their practice.

Presumably as a direct result of removing a greater volume of lung tissue, bilateral LVRS results in a greater short-term physiological improvement than unilateral surgery.[6] A bilateral approach, however, is associated with a faster decline in forced expiratory volume (FEV_1). A staged unilateral approach therefore may not only reduce the operative risk but also prolong the benefits of LVRS. The first lung to be reduced usually will be the one with least perfusion on quantitative radionuclide scintigraphy. If the distribution is relatively equal, then the larger right lung is reduced first.

The timing of the second side operation may be determined by the surgeon based on an assessment of the patient's recovery from the initial operation. The subsequent operative risk then may be reduced. The authors favor a decision on the timing of the second operation made in conjunction with the patient. Based on the rationale that LVRS is primarily an operation to improve the subjective sensation of breathlessness rather than achieve objective improvements in FEV_1, the authors prefer to allow the patient to decide when he or she would like to have further surgery. This decision is based on his or her assessment of symptoms of dyspnea and his or her exercise capacity. Once the timing of the contralateral LVRS has been agreed upon, repeat preoperative physiological and anatomical assessments are made.

The authors' patients are aware from the outset that LVRS is not a cure for their emphysema. Rather LVRS is a means of temporarily reversing their natural decline into disability by pushing them back up a virtual slope. They are aware that they will continue to slide down the slope postoperatively as their emphysema progresses. A staged approach to LVRS allows them a second chance to be pushed back up the slope.

Department of Thoracic Surgery, Glenfield Hospital, UHL-NHS Trust, Groby Road, Leicester LE3 9QP, UK
* Corresponding author.
E-mail address: david.waller@uhl-tr.nhs.uk (D. Waller).

Thorac Surg Clin 19 (2009) 187–192
doi:10.1016/j.thorsurg.2009.02.001

EXPERIENCE
Unilateral or Bilateral Surgery?

There is a lack of randomized clinical evidence comparing these two strategies, but there are a small number of clinical series indirectly comparing the outcome from these different approaches.

Kotloff and colleagues[6] compared the short-term functional outcomes following LVRS performed unilaterally in 32 patients and bilaterally in 119 patients. Bilateral LVRS was associated with increased in-hospital mortality (10% versus 0%, $P<.05$) and a higher incidence of postoperative respiratory failure (12.6% versus 0%; $P<.05$) compared with unilateral LVRS. There was no significant difference in duration of air leaks between unilateral and bilateral groups, but the mean hospital stay was significantly longer following bilateral LVRS (21.1 plus or minus 32.0 days versus 14.2 plus or minus 14.0 days; $P<.05$). The magnitude of improvement in each physiological parameter following unilateral LVRS exceeded half that following bilateral LVRS, suggesting that functional outcomes after the unilateral procedure were disproportionate to the amount of tissue resected. Only seven patients underwent staged unilateral procedures (two unilateral procedures separated in time by at least 3 months) and demonstrated somewhat unpredictable responses. The authors concluded that unilateral LVRS should be reserved for patients in whom factors contraindicating entrance into one hemithorax exist.

Serna and colleagues[7] compared the 2-year survival of 260 patients who underwent unilateral versus bilateral video-assisted LVRS in a large cohort treated by a single surgical group. Overall survival at 2 years was 86.4% (95% CI 80.9% to 91.8%) after bilateral LVRS versus 72.6% (95% CI 64.2% to 81.2%) after unilateral LVRS ($P = .001$ for overall survival comparison). Improved survival after bilateral LVRS was seen among high- and low-risk subgroups also. Average follow-up time was 28.5 months (range, 6 days to 46.6 months) for the bilateral LVRS group and 29.3 months (range, 6 days to 45.0 months) for the unilateral LVRS patients. Bilateral LVRS by VATS resulted in better overall survival at 2-year follow-up than did unilateral LVRS. On the basis of this evidence, the authors concluded that bilateral surgery appears to be the procedure of choice for patients undergoing LVRS for most eligible patients who have severe heterogeneous emphysema. They failed to acknowledge that the two groups were not comparable in that not all the unilateral patients had bilateral target areas. They probably had homogenous, more advanced emphysema with a worse intrinsic prognosis.

In an article by Oey and colleagues[3] of the Glenfield experience, the authors compared the long-term physiological and health status outcome of LVRS performed on one or simultaneously on both lungs in a consecutive series of 65 patients undergoing LVRS who were all suitable for bilateral surgery. Twenty-six patients aged 57.5 (8) years underwent bilateral LVRS by VATS or sternotomy and 39 patients aged 60 ($\pm$6) years underwent unilateral VATS. Unilateral LVRS was associated with significantly lower weight of lung resected (80 [$\pm$31] versus 118 [$\pm$46] g) and shorter length of hospital stay (16 [$\pm$10] days versus 28 [$\pm$22] days). There was no significant difference in 30-day mortality, but postoperative ventilation was more common in the bilateral group (5% in the unilateral versus 42% in the bilateral group [$P = .0002$]). The decline of FEV_1 during the first postoperative year was significant in the bilateral group (-313 mL/y, $P = .04$) but not significant in the unilateral group (-50 mL/y, $P = .18$). SF 36 scores in all eight domains were similar in both groups preoperatively and at any postoperative interval.

The authors have found no benefit from bilateral simultaneous LVRS and prefer unilateral LVRS because of the lower morbidity, resulting in earlier discharge and slower decline in physiological benefit.

In the Edinburgh experience, staged unilateral VATS with a 9-month interval did not improve significantly on the physiological results of the first operation.[8] The overall benefits, however, were prolonged by 1 year. LVRS was performed as a unilateral VATS procedure, with bilateral reduction being undertaken in a staged manner. Twenty-one patients had staged reduction of the contralateral lung at a median interval of 9 months. Preoperatively, patients undergoing sequential LVR were not significantly different from 29 patients undergoing unilateral LVR. After single-side LVR, both groups demonstrated equivalent and significant improvement in spirometric and subjective health scores (FEV_1 + 15% predicted [$P<.01$], TLC -5% [$P = .03$], health score +80% [$P<.01$]). Patients undergoing sequential reduction demonstrated no further significant improvements using either an intragroup comparison with their presecond operation values or an intergroup comparison with the unilateral LVR patients. Sequential LVR, however, appeared to prolong the benefits experienced after the initial surgery by 1 year. Overall, 12 patients (24%) died during follow-up, with no survival difference between the two groups ($P = .65$). Undertaking LVR to the second side was not found to improve spirometric or subjective performance but did prolong the benefits achieved with the initial reduction.

Pompeo[9] compared a one-stage versus a two-stage bilateral approach at the reappearance of symptoms.[8] Fifty-nine patients undergoing bilateral thoracoscopic reduction pneumoplasty as a one-stage (n = 33) or staged (n = 26) procedure were evaluated. The main indication for staged reduction pneumoplasty was symptom deterioration after unilateral treatment for asymmetric emphysema. The mean length of follow-up was 34 plus or minus15 months. Interval time between operations in the staged group averaged 15.2 months. Peak improvements in FEV_1, forced vital capacity (FVC), and residual volume (RV) were significantly greater following one-stage bilateral reduction pneumoplasty. At 48 months, FEV_1, RV and 6-minute walking-test (6MWT) remained significantly improved only in the staged group. Four-year survival was not significantly different between the groups. Durable physiological improvements and satisfactory survival were achieved in this study for up to 4 years following either staged or one-stage VATS bilateral reduction pneumoplasty. Although peak improvements in FEV_1, FVC, and RV were significantly greater following one-stage bilateral reduction, however, long-term improvements in FVC and 6MWT were more stable following a staged procedure. The authors suggested that sequential unilateral LVRS may reduce the mechanical stress in the lung leading to less steep postoperative deterioration of respiratory function.

In the authors' current experience of 81 patients treated with the intent of staged bilateral LVRS, only 15 patients have proceeded to the second operation. The median time between operations is currently 4 years, ranging from 9 months to over 6 years. Of the 66 patients who have not proceeded to the second stage, 31 remain undecided; 24 have died, and 11 have deteriorated below selection criteria with falls in FEV_1 and DLCO.

In their series, Pompeo and Mineo[9] noted that only 31% of those who underwent an initial unilateral operation required completion of bilateral treatment. Allowing for a small number of patients who died and a smaller number who declined, most had sustained benefit for up to 4 years after their first operation.

The question arises, "Why do these patients not request surgery at an earlier stage?"

A few patients will not have received any benefit form their first operation and so will not be considered for more LVRS. In most, however, the benefit from unilateral LVRS has been more durable than expected.

UNILATERAL LUNG VOLUME REDUCTION SURGERY MAY BE ALL THAT IS REQUIRED

The authors observed in a population of 77 patients, including 47 unilateral LVRS cases, that the changes in FEV_1 are only significantly improved for 1 year after LVRS, while the improvements in TLC and RV remain significant up to 3 years postoperatively.[9] The improvements in body mass index (BMI) also persist for 3 years. The best scores in Euroquol and SF 36 are obtained 6 months after LVRS but only are improved significantly up to 1 year. The physiological effects of unilateral LVRS appear to be lasting, but initial improvements in health status decline more rapidly. The authors also have found that postoperative pain detracts from global improvement in health status after LVRS even after unilateral VATS. There may be an influence of alterations in chest mechanics after surgery on the development of pain.[11] In 52 patients, after unilateral LVRS, significant improvements in health status—as assessed by SF 36—persisted from 3 months to 1 year. In the pain domain, however, there was a worsening of the mean score for between 40% and 45% of patients even 2 years after LVRS. Other authors have also documented objective improvements in physiological parameters and health status assessments,[12,13] but these benefits are not durable and last for between 2 and 3 years.

The authors additionally have found an overall increase in BMI after LVRS, which was significant up to 2 years. These changes correlated with the changes in FEV1 (R = 0.3, $P<.01$ 6 months after LVRS); diffusing capacity for carbon monoxide (DLCO) (R = 0.5, $P<.01$ 6 months after LVRS), and reflected changes in health status.[14] The perioperative course of LVRS and its physiological benefits are influenced by preoperative BMI. Postoperative physiological improvements in the first year were related to preoperative BMI for FEV_1 (R = 0.29, P = .02) and DLCO (R = 0.33, P = .02). Postoperative BMI significantly increased in the underweight yet significantly decreased in the overweight at all time points. Although the treatment of the underweight is more complicated, LVRS may be the only way of increasing their BMI.[15]

Some patients therefore may be so satisfied with their improvement after unilateral LVRS that they never need to request a contralateral operation. For the surgeon, there may be a tendency to remove more lung if only operating on one side. Furthermore the concern about persistent air leak or apical space may be lessened if the contralateral lung is left untouched.

WHAT FACTORS DETERMINE THE TIMING OF THE SECOND SIDE OPERATION?

The second side operation may be unplanned and dictated by technical factors. Such factors include patient instability from a large unilateral air leak,[9] which may lead to the abandonment of a planned bilateral operation. The second side then may require rescheduling. The operation may preplanned by the surgeon. Once the patient has recovered from the first side, he or she may advise proceeding to the second operation immediately. The operation may be preplanned for a set interval, calculated from previous results, when physiological improvement is at its peak (around 12 months) as suggested by Soon.[8] This would be intended to retard the decline in objective physiological parameters, including FEV_1.

The timing of the second side operation may be unplanned from the outset and determined by variable factors. The operation may be timed for the first sign in physiological decline as measured by spirometry on regular follow-up examinations. This method has the attraction of being patient-based, but physiological parameters may vary depending on other factors (ie, concurrent infection). The authors prefer the patient to make the decision based on his or her subjective assessment of symptoms supported by objective health status questionnaires.

HEALTH STATUS

Several authors have noted that postoperative benefits in health status parameters continue long after improvements in physiological measures have declined. Others have noted that there is no clear correlation between spirometric improvements and changes in health status.[16] A staged

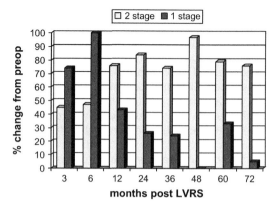

Fig. 2. The effect of operative strategy on postoperative change in the social functioning domain of the SF36 health status questionnaire.

bilateral approach has been shown to have more durable benefits in health status than a one-stop operation. Mineo reported improvement in physical functioning for more than 4 years after LVRS overall but for up to 6 years in only the staged bilateral group.[17] The authors' preliminary results in the relatively small numbers of their population who have undergone their second operation suggest that that this second interventions reverses the decline in specific health status indicators. In the domains of the SF-36 tool concerning social and physical functioning and energy/vitality, previous reports have shown significant improvements up to 2 years after bilateral LVRS, effects that were attributable more to surgery than preoperative rehabilitation.[18,19] The authors have found a steady decline in the follow-up measurements of health status after one-stage bilateral LVRS. They, however, have noticed a second-wave increase in these variables following the completion of the sequential

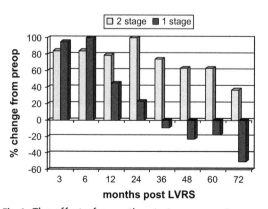

Fig. 1. The effect of operative strategy on postoperative change in the physical functioning domain of the SF36 health status questionnaire.

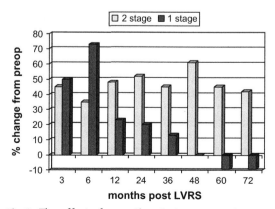

Fig. 3. The effect of operative strategy on postoperative change in the energy/vitality domain of the SF36 health status questionnaire.

treatment. The improvements in the single-stage patients lasted up to 12 months, whereas in the staged bilateral group, the improvements in these domains lasted for up to 5 years (**Figs. 1–3**).

SURVIVAL

LVRS is associated with improved survival over maximal medical treatment in certain clinical groups of patients who have chronic obstructive pulmonary disease (COPD). There is little evidence to suggest that the surgical strategy influences overall survival. Mineo reported 5-year actuarial survival of 88% and 77% after two- stage and one-stage LVRS respectively with no significant difference.[10] The experience from Edinburgh[8] is that a policy of sequential LVRS does not result in any additional risk, with a 4-year mortality rate of around 20% to 25%, which does not differ significantly from large series of one-stage bilateral surgery.[20] The authors have found no difference in 3- or 5-year survival between those who have had one-stage bilateral and those who have had staged surgery; 5-year survival approached 60% in both groups.

WHAT ARE THE POTENTIAL PROBLEMS WITH A STAGED BILATERAL APPROACH?

Patients may die of their underlying lung disease or its complications before being assessed for the second operation. A one-stage bilateral approach may increase overall survival in this population suitable for LVRS. There is a distinct possibility that some patients may deteriorate physiologically even though their symptoms may be acceptable. Then by the time they decide that they need further surgery they are no longer suitable. This problem may be avoided by regular follow-up examinations including health status assessment.

The main reason, however, why a one-stage bilateral approach to LVRS is considered to be the standard of care[21] (certainly in the United States) appears to be financial. Hazelrigg[22] found no measurable advantages in a staged approach in terms of short-term morbidity or functional results. The costs of two separate procedures and hospital episodes became prohibitive. It would appear that short-term benefits rather than the long-term health status benefits have shaped surgical policy. The more conservative surgeons remain in the minority. The message that a staged bilateral LVRS can lead to a more sustained benefit with a second wind in well being is not accepted widely. Not everyone has understood the fable of the tortoise and the hare.

REFERENCES

1. Brantigan O, Mueller E. Surgical treatment of pulmonary emphysema. Am Surg 1957;23:789–804.
2. Cooper JD, Trulock EP, Triantafillou AN, et al. Bilateral pneumectomy for chronic obstructive pulmonary disease. J Thorac Cardiovasc Surg 1995;109:106–16.
3. Oey I, Waller DA, Bal S, et al. Lung volume reduction surgery—a comparison of the long-term outcome of unilateral vs bilateral approaches. Eur J Cardiothorac Surg 2002;22(4):610–4.
4. National Emphysema Treatment Trial Research Group. Safety and efficacy of median sternotomy versus video-assisted thoracic surgery for lung volume reduction surgery. J Thorac Cardiovasc Surg 2004;127:1350–60.
5. Brenner M, McKenna RJ, Gelb AF, et al. Rate of FEV1 change following lung volume reduction surgery. Chest 1998;113:652–9.
6. Kotloff RM, Tino G, Bavaria JE, et al. Comparison of short-term functional outcomes following unilateral and bilateral lung volume reduction surgery. Chest 1998;113(4):890–5.
7. Serna DL, Brenner M, Osann KE, et al. Survival after unilateral versus bilateral lung volume reduction surgery for emphysema. J Thorac Cardiovasc Surg 1999;118(6):1101–9.
8. Soon SY, Saidi G, Ong ML, et al. Sequential VATS lung volume reduction surgery: prolongation of benefits derived after the initial operation. Eur J Cardiothorac Surg 2003 Jul;24(1):149–53.
9. Pompeo E, Mineo TC, Pulmonary Emphysema Research Group. Long-term outcome of staged versus one-stage bilateral thoracoscopic reduction pneumoplasty. Eur J Cardiothorac Surg 2002;21(4):627–33.
10. Oey I, Morgan MD, Singh SJ, et al. The long-term health status improvements seen after lung volume reduction surgery. Eur J Cardiothorac Surg 2003;24(4):614–9.
11. Oey I, Morgan MD, Waller DA. Postoperative pain detracts from early health status improvement seen after video-assisted thoracoscopic lung volume reduction surgery. Eur J Cardiothorac Surg 2003;24(4):588–93.
12. Geiser T, Schwizer B, Krueger T, et al. Outcome after unilateral lung volume reduction surgery in patients with severe emphysema. Eur J Cardiothorac Surg 2001;20:674–8.
13. Meyers BF, Sultan PK, Guthrie TJ, et al. Outcomes after unilateral lung volume reduction. Ann Thorac Surg 2008;86:204–11.
14. Oey I, Waller DA, Bal S, et al. The increase in body mass index observed after lung volume reduction may act as surrogate marker of improved health status. Respir Med 2004;98(3):247–53.
15. Vaughan P, Oey I, Steiner MC, et al. A prospective analysis of the inter-relationship between lung volume reduction surgery and body mass index. Eur J Cardiothorac Surg 2007;32(6):839–42.

16. Leyenson V, Furukawa S, Kuzma A, et al. Correlation of changes in quality of life after LVRS with changes in lung function, exercise, and gas exchange. Chest 2000;118:728–35.

17. Mineo TC, Pompeo E. Long-term results of tailored lung volume reduction surgery for severe emphysema. Clin Ter 2007;158:127–33.

18. Hamacher J, Buchi S, Georgescu CL, et al. Improved quality of life after lung volume reduction surgery. Eur Respir J 2002;19:54–60.

19. Moy ML, Ingenito EP, Mentzer SJ, et al. Health-related quality of life improves following pulmonary rehabilitation and lung volume reduction surgery. Chest 1999;115:383–9.

20. Cooper JD, Lefrak SS. LVR: 5 years on. Lancet 1999; 353(Suppl 1):26–7.

21. DeCamp MM, McKenna RJ, Deschamps CC, et al. Lung volume reduction surgery: technique, operative mortality, and morbidity. Proc Am Thorac Soc 2008;5:442–6.

22. Hazelrigg SR, Boley TM, Magee MJ, et al. Comparison of staged thoracoscopy and median sternotomy for lung volume reduction. Ann Thorac Surg 1998;66: 1134–9.

Lung Volume Reduction Surgery in Nonheterogeneous Emphysema

Walter Weder, MD[a],*, Michaela Tutic, MD[a], Konrad E. Bloch, MD[b]

KEYWORDS

- Homogeneous emphysema
- Lung volume reduction surgery • Bullae
- Hyperinflation • Pulmonary mechanics

Lung volume reduction surgery (LVRS) is an established, successful, palliative surgical therapy for carefully selected patients with advanced emphysema. Although the experience with LVRS has grown over the last few years, the selection of patients suitable for LVRS is still a matter of major controversy and differs widely between centers. On the basis of the early work from Brantigen[1] and that was revived by Cooper,[2] the procedure was recommended to be performed as a nonanatomic resection of the most severely destroyed, functionless tissue to reduce lung volume by 20% to 30%. Patients with a homogeneous type of emphysema were not considered suitable for LVRS. Most centers exclusively selected patients with a heterogeneous emphysema, preferentially located in the upper lobes as assessed by CT scans or by perfusion scintigraphy.

The mechanisms of action of LVRS relate mainly to changes in respiratory mechanics. The reduction in hyperinflation results in an increase in elastic recoil of the lungs, which reduces airflow obstruction and restores the chest cavity, including the shape of the diaphragm, thereby improving its length-tension relationship. These effects have a positive impact on shortness of breath, quality of life,[3,4] lung function and exercise capacity as shown in several prospective single-center case studies[5–7] and a few randomized, controlled trials.[8–12] Particularly, the results of the large national emphysema treatment trial (NETT) confirmed that properly selected patients

may experience better functional improvements and quality of life after surgery than with medical treatment. This was especially the case for patients with upper lobe predominant destruction of the lungs and a poor exercise capacity. The trial did not exclude, but also did not support the fact that patients with homogeneous emphysema may also benefit from LVRS since only a few patients with such morphology were included in the NETT. In most centers, patients who did not show heterogeneity as the emphysematous destruction seen on CT were either excluded from surgery or thought to experience only minor benefits. In these patients, distinct areas of non- or poorly perfused lung could not be identified on perfusion scans as targets for resection, and they were, therefore, not considered candidates for LVRS. Since the favorable effects of LVRS are mainly caused by the improvement of respiratory mechanics, we postulated that well-selected patients with severe hyperinflation and airflow obstruction should benefit in dyspnea, quality of life, lung function, and physical performance, even if their emphysema was nonheterogeneously distributed.

RATIONALE OF LUNG VOLUME REDUCTION SURGERY IN HETEROGENEOUS AND NONHETEROGENEOUS EMPHYSEMA

The pathophysiological mechanisms responsible for improvements after LVRS are multifactorious

a Department of Surgery, Division of Thoracic Surgery, University Hospital, Zurich, Raemistrasse 100, 8091 Zürich, Switzerland
b Pulmonary Division, University Hospital, Zurich, Raemistrasse 100, CH- 8091 Zürich, Switzerland
* Corresponding author.
E-mail address: walter.weder@usz.ch (W. Weder).

Thorac Surg Clin 19 (2009) 193–199
doi:10.1016/j.thorsurg.2009.03.002
1547-4127/09/$ – see front matter © 2009 Elsevier Inc. All rights reserved.

and still not fully understood. The major early effects of LVRS are a reduction in static lung volumes, particularly functional residual capacity and residual volume (RV), associated with an increase in lung elastic recoil, which leads to a reduction in the degree of airflow obstruction and hyperinflation, and hence, a reduced work of breathing. Measurements of elastic recoil before and after LVRS support this assumption. In 20 subjects undergoing LVRS, 16 experienced an increase in elastic recoil.[13] These patients had a significantly greater improvement in exercise capacity than those in whom elastic recoil didn't change. In addition to its effects on respiratory mechanics, LVRS improves global inspiratory muscle strength[14–17] and the contribution of the diaphragm to inspiratory pressure generation and tidal volume both at rest and during exercise.[18,19] Thus, by decreasing respiratory muscle load and by increasing diaphragmatic strength, LVRS enhances diaphragmatic neuromechanical coupling.[17] Since LVRS makes the diaphragmatic dome move upward and increases the area of muscle apposed to the rib cage,[20] it reduces dyspnea, and improves maximal ventilatory and exercise capacity by optimizing the match between size of the lungs and the rib cage.[21] These effects are independent from the emphysema morphology, and therefore, patients with homogeneous emphysema should also benefit from LVRS. There have been concerns that in patients with homogeneous emphysema who undergo LVRS, parenchyma contributing to gas exchange will be resected. This disadvantage of surgery has to be compensated by a beneficiary effect of downsizing the hyperinflated lung to a more physiologic size.

THE ROLE OF EMPHYSEMA MORPHOLOGY IN LUNG VOLUME REDUCTION SURGERY

Emphysema is defined anatomically. In its severe form it can be easily detected on a plain posteroanterior and lateral chest radiograph. However, the most reliable method of obtaining information on the degree and distribution of emphysema is chest CT scanning. This imaging method plays a major role in the selection process. It is obvious that LVRS would be particularly beneficial in patients with a heterogeneous distribution of emphysematous destruction, such as in patients with large bullae beside areas that are well preserved. Earlier experience with bullectomy in patients with emphysema supported such a concept. Most groups, especially in North America,[6,22] preferentially select patients with marked differences in the severity of emphysema in their lung. They argue that these areas are functionless and should be chosen as target areas for resection. However, a few European groups have also operated on patients with completely a homogeneus distribution pattern of emphysema[23–25] and have studied this concept prospectively.

Different morphologic grading systems have been developed to quantify the type, severity, and distribution of emphysema as a help in identifying candidates for LVRS, although no internationally accepted standardized radiological classification exists. Slone and Gierada[26] based their analysis on a sophisticated classification system of emphysema morphology that showed good correlations with functional outcome. Favorable radiological features included marked heterogeneity of emphysema, particularly upper lobe predominance accompanied by mildly affected lung areas, and the presence of compressed lung. This classification system was modified by Wisser and colleagues[27] to achieve a higher degree of reproducibility and a mathematical quantification of heterogeneity and severity of disease. The morphology of emphysema was quantified using standard chest radiographs and CT imaging on the basis of four variables: degree of hyperinflation, degree of impairment in diaphragmatic mechanics, degree of heterogeneity, and severity of parenchymal destruction. Other authors have concluded from qualitative visual analysis of the chest radiography, from the CT or quantitative CT densitometry,[28,29] or from analysis of perfusion scans,[30] that emphysema heterogeneity indicates favorable outcome. A specifically LVRS oriented classification system based on CT findings was proposed by Weder and colleagues[31,32] distinguishing between homogeneous, moderately heterogeneous, and markedly heterogeneous emphysema distribution, and the predominance of the involved side was considered. The following definitions were applied (**Fig. 1**): Markedly heterogeneous emphysema occurs when a distinct regional difference in the severity of emphysema (ie, decreased density, loss of vascular lung structure) is present in at least two adjacent lung segments of either lung. Intermediately heterogeneous emphysema occurs when a distinct regional difference in severity of emphysema may be present maximally in the area of one or more than one, but not in adjacent lung segments of either lung. Markedly heterogeneous emphysema occurs when a distinct regional difference in the severity of emphysema is present in at least the area of two adjacent lung segments of either lung. This classification system is easy to apply, helps to select patients for LVRS, and allows comparison of outcome.

Markedly **Heterogeneous**

upper lobe   upper lobe and apical segment (lower lobe)   lower lobe (basal segment)

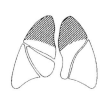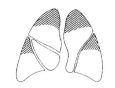

Intermediately **Heterogeneous**

anatomically indistinct   anatomically distinct (lower lobe)

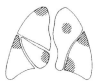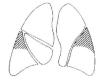

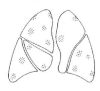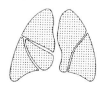

Homogeneous

with patchy areas   completely homogeneous

Fig. 1. Classification system of emphysema. Three major types of emphysema distribution were defined: markedly heterogeneous (*upper panel*), intermediately heterogeneous (*middle panel*), and homogeneous (*lower panel*). For heterogeneous emphysema types, the most affected areas were recorded as disease predominance in either upper lobe, upper lobe and apical segment of the lower lobe, or lower lobe. Among homogeneous types of emphysema (*lower panel*) some showed multiple small zones of destruction throughout all lobes (patchy). In other emphysematous changes were evenly distributed throughout the entire lungs (homogeneous). (*From* Weder W, Thurnheer R, Stammberger U, et al. Radiologic emphysema morphology is associated with outcome after surgical lung volume reduction. Ann Thorac Surg 1997; 64(2):314; with permission.)

SURGICAL APPROACH AND DEFINITION OF THE TARGET AREA FOR RESECTION

LVRS is typically performed under general anesthesia, during one lung ventilation by way of median sternotomy, thoracotomy or bilateral video-assisted thoracoscopic surgery. It can be performed uni- or bilaterally. The target areas and the extent of resection differs between various types of emphysema. The lung is resected in areas that show the most severe emphysematous destruction on imaging studies (CT scan) corresponding to a loss of perfusion on quantitative perfusion scan (heterogeneous type).[33] This is either in the upper lobes or the basal segments of the lower lobes. Some patients have a combination of upper lobe (apical) and lower lobe (apical segment) destruction. In those patients approximately 30% to 40% of the upper lobe is resected, in combination with the apical segment of the lower lobe. In patients with homogenous emphysema it is more difficult to define the amount and site of resection since clearly defined target areas are absent. In these cases we preferentially choose the upper lobes for resection. The amount of resection is approximately 40% to 50% of the upper lobes, which is the volume needed to reduce the total lung capacity to the predicted volume. Since the resected volume cannot be quantified during surgery, the ideal volume of resection cannot be assessed scientifically.

The selection criteria should be applied very strictly in patients with homogeneous destruction. The only valuable candidates for LVRS are patients with severe hyperinflation in absence of pulmonary hypertension, with no signs of recurrent infections or purulent bronchitis, and with a diffusing capacity not less than 20% predicted, which is especially important.

RESULTS OF SURGERY OF NONHETEROGENEOUS EMPHYSEMA

Only very limited published studies are available on the effect of LVRS in homogenous emphysema.[23,25,31] Wisser and colleagues have reported short-term outcome of 54 patients with homogeneous emphysema between 1994 and 1996; whereas, Weder and coworkers in Zurich have studied 138 patients with homogeneous destruction of the lung undergoing LVRS between 1994 and 2008 in comparison with other morphologies, and described the outcome over several years.[25] Other groups did not report on data on patients with homogeneous emphysema.

DYSPNEA

LVRS considerably improved dyspnea in the homogeneous group, where the Medical Research Council score decreased by 1.6 points from 3.46 (±0.7) to 1.8 (±0.9) (P<.001) after LVRS and remained below baseline for up to 4 years. In the heterogeneous group it decreased by 2.1 points from 3.47 (±0.7) to 1.3 (±0.9) (P<.001) after LVRS and remained significantly decreased for up to 5 years.

PULMONARY FUNCTION AND GAS EXCHANGE

Three months after LVRS, the Zurich group found relevant symptomatic and functional improvements in heterogeneous and in homogenous emphysema

(**Fig. 2**). Maximal values were observed 3 to 6 months after operation with a subsequent decline toward preoperative levels over the following years.[34]

In 138 subjects with homogeneous emphysema FEV_1 increased by 35% from 0.70 (±0.19) L (27.6±7.2% predicted) to 0.95 (±0.34) L (38±14% predicted) (P<.001) 3 months after LVRS. TLC decreased from 7.77 (±1.5) L to 7.14 (±1.4) L and RV decreased from 5.31 (±1.3) L to 4.15 (±1.07) L at 3 months after LVRS (P<.001) resulting in a reduction of the RV/TLC ratio from 0.68 (±0.07) to 0.58 (±0.08) (P<.001) in the homogeneous group, whereas in 121 patients who had heterogeneous emphysema, the FEV_1 increased by 61% from 0.78 (±0.25) L (27.9+8.5 % predicted) to 1.26 (±0.53) L (44+15 % predicted) (p<0.001) and the RV/TLC ratio decreased from 0.67 (±0.09) to 0.52 (±0.11) (p<0.001) 3 months after LVRS.[25] The beneficial effect on hyperinflation remained statistically significant for up to two years in both groups (see **Fig. 2**).

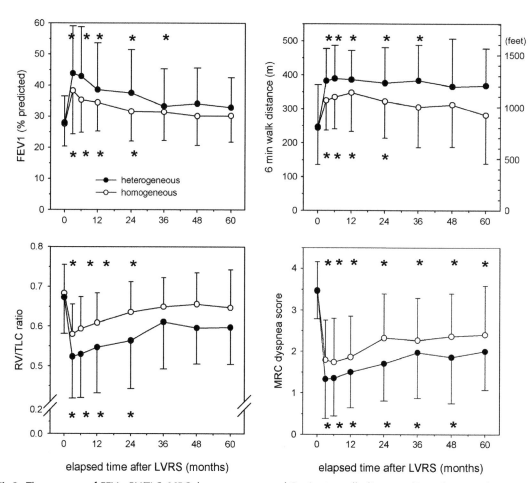

Fig 2. Time course of FEV_1, RV/TLC, MRC dyspnea score, and 6-minute walk distance. (*Data from* Weder W, Tutic M, Lardinois D, et al. Persistent benefit from lung volume reduction surgery in patients with homogeneous emphysema. Ann Thorac Surg 2009;87(1):229–36.)

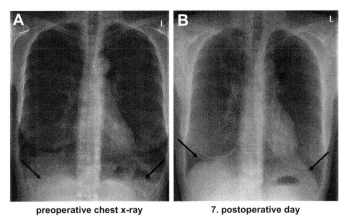

preoperative chest x-ray   7. postoperative day

Fig. 3. (*A*) Preoperative chest radiograph. (*B*) 7-day postoperative.

Fig. 3 illustrates the effect of LVRS on the radiograph in a patient with homogeneous emphysema. The preoperative severe hyperinflation of the lung with the depressed and flattened diaphragm is postoperatively diminished; it is visible in the regain of the clear dome shape of the diaphragm. Independent of the emphysema morphology, the values of FEV_1 and the 6-minute walking distance return to values near baseline after a median period of 36 months (see **Fig. 2**), although patients perceive persistent improvements in dyspnea for a much longer time (ie, for 4–5 years).

The PaO_2 increased from 64.4 ($\pm$8.2) mmHg to 67.4 ($\pm$8.3) mmHg and remained above baseline for up to 6 months ($P<.01$), while the mean $PaCO_2$ decreased from 40.1 ($\pm$5.4) mmHg to 37.8 ($\pm$4.6) mmHg and remained lower than preoperatively for up to 12 months ($P<.05$) even in the homogeneous group.

SURVIVAL

The overall perioperative mortality in LVRS is low (Wieser: 1.2%; Weder: <1%) and the BODE index significantly increases suggesting a positive survival effect.[35]

We observed similar survival curves in patients with homogeneous and heterogeneous emphysema, in the perioperative period and up to 1 year (**Fig. 4**). But subsequently, patients with heterogeneous emphysema had a slightly better chance of surviving without lung transplantation than patients with homogeneous emphysema. The hazard ratio of patients with heterogeneous versus homogeneous emphysema was 0.81 (95% CI, 0.66–0.98, P = .03) when controlling for potential confounders including age, gender, body mass index, alpha1 antitrypsin deficiency, baseline FEV_1, RV/TLC ratio, diffusing capacity, MRC score, and 6-minute walk distance.

An unacceptably high mortality in a subgroup of NETT subjects resulted in an early press release of a widely noted article in the New England Journal of Medicine.[36] For 69 subjects who had an FEV_1 no more than 20% of predicted, and either a homogeneous distribution of emphysema or a carbon monoxide diffusing capacity less than 20% of predicted, the 30-day mortality rate after surgery was 16%, compared to a rate of 0% among 70 medically treated subjects ($P<.001$). Most experienced centers have excluded such patients from surgery from the beginning of their LVRS program since they expected such a dismal outcome when lung reduction is performed in patients with uniformly destroyed (vanished) lung.

SUMMARY

Patients with a homogeneous type of emphysema have been excluded a priori from LVRS in many

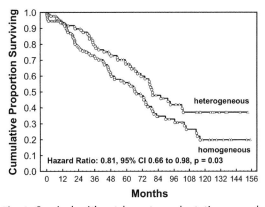

Fig. 4. Survival without lung transplantation according to emphysema morphology. (*Data from* Weder W, Tutic M, Lardinois D, et al. Persistent benefit from lung volume reduction surgery in patients with homogeneous emphysema. Ann Thorac Surg 2009; 87(1):229–36.)

centers because of the fear of removing parenchyma, which potentially contributes to gas exchange, and because the observation that heterogeneity of emphysema is a predictor of functional improvement. It is obvious that resection of functionless tissue, such as in heterogeneous emphysema with bullae, can be advised to the patient with a relative low risk. However, as the main positive effect of LVRS is its improvement on respiratory mechanics, it is not surprising that well-selected patients with homogeneous emphysema also benefit from surgery. Their selection has to be done cautiously. It is crucial to exclude patients with a very low functional reserve, such as with diffusing capacity below 20% predicted or with pulmonary hypertension, and with extreme parenchymal loss (vanished lungs) on CT from LVRS. Additionally, cofactors which may potentially interfere with a smooth postoperative course, such as previous recurrent infections, extensive scarring of the lungs, or previous surgery, have to be taken into consideration. When respecting these caveats, LVRS in patients with complete homogeneous emphysema provides a comparable symptomatic and almost the same functional improvement as in patients with heterogeneous emphysema. Although the perioperative mortality is low, patients with homogeneous emphysema have a slightly reduced long-term survival without lung transplantation compared with patients with heterogeneous emphysema. Based on our own experience, we conclude that LVRS can be recommended to selected symptomatic patients with advanced homogenous emphysema associated with severe hyperinflation, if diffusing capacity is not below 20% of predicted values and if the CT scan does not show aspects of vanished lungs.

REFERENCES

1. Brantigan OC, Kress MB, Mueller EA. The surgical approach to pulmonary emphysema. Dis Chest 1961;39:485–501.
2. Cooper JD, Patterson GA, Sundaresan RS, et al. Results of 150 consecutive bilateral lung volume reduction procedures in patients with severe emphysema. J Thorac Cardiovasc Surg 1996;112(5):1319–30.
3. Hamacher J, Buchi S, Georgescu CL, et al. Improved quality of life after lung volume reduction surgery. Eur Respir J 2002;19(1):54–60.
4. Martinez FJ, Montes de Oca M, Whyte RI, et al. Lung-volume reduction improves dyspnea, dynamic hyperinflation, and respiratory muscle function. Am J Respir Crit Care Med 1997;155:1984–90.
5. Gelb AF, McKenna RJ Jr, Brenner M, et al. Lung function 5 yr after lung volume reduction surgery for emphysema. Am J Respir Crit Care Med 2001; 163(7):1562–6.
6. Ciccone AM, Meyers BF, Guthrie TJ, et al. Long-term outcome of bilateral lung volume reduction in 250 consecutive patients with emphysema. J Thorac Cardiovasc Surg 2003;125(3):513–25.
7. Fujimoto T, Teschler H, Hillejan L, et al. Long-term results of lung volume reduction surgery. Eur J Cardiothorac Surg 2002;21(3):483–8.
8. Criner GJ, Cordova FC, Furukawa S, et al. Prospective randomized trial comparing bilateral lungvolume reduction surgery to pulmonary rehabilitation in severe chronic obstructive pulmonary disease. Am J Respir Crit Care Med 1999;160(6):2018–27.
9. Miller J, Berger R, Malthaner R. Lung volume reduction surgery vs. medical treatment: for patients with advanced emphysema. Chest 2005;127:1166–77.
10. Cleverley JR, Desai SR, Wells AU, et al. Evaluation of patients undergoing lung volume reduction surgery: ancillary information available from computed tomography. Clin Radiol 2000;55(1):45–50.
11. Pompeo E, Marino M, Nofroni I, et al. Reduction pneumoplasty versus respiratory rehabilitation in severe emphysema: a randomized study. Pulmonary Emphysema Research Group. Ann Thorac Surg 2000;70(3):948–53.
12. NETT. Cost effectiveness of lung-volume-reduction surgery for patients with severe emphysema. N Engl J Med 2003;348(21):2092–102.
13. Sciurba FC, Rogers RM, Keenan RJ, et al. Improvement in pulmonary function and elastic recoil after lung-reduction surgery for diffuse emphysema. N Engl J Med 1996;334(17):1095–9.
14. O'Donnell DE, Webb KA, Bertley J, et al. Mechanisms of relief of exertional breathlessness following unilateral bullectomy and lung volume reduction surgery in emphysema. Chest 1996;110(1):18–27.
15. Teschler H, Stamatis G, El-Raouf Farhat AA, et al. Effect of surgical lung volume reduction on respiratory muscle function in pulmonary emphysema. Eur Respir J 1996;9:1779–84.
16. Lando Y, Boiselle PM, Shade D, et al. Effect of lung volume reduction surgery on diaphragm length in severe chronic obstructive pulmonary disease. Am J Respir Crit Care Med 1999;159(3):796–805.
17. Laghi F, Jubran A, Topeli A, et al. Effect of lung volume reduction surgery on neuromechanical coupling of the diaphragm. Am J Respir Crit Care Med 1998;157(2):475–83.
18. Bloch KE, Li Y, Zhang J, et al. Effect of surgical lung volume reduction on breathing patterns in severe pulmonary emphysema. Am J Respir Crit Care Med 1997;156:553–60.
19. Benditt J, Wood DE, McCool FD, et al. Changes in breathing and ventilatory muscle recruitment patterns induced by lung volume reduction surgery. Am J Respir Crit Care Med 1997;155(1):279–84.

20. Cassart M, Hamacher J, Verbandt Y, et al. Effects of lung volume reduction surgery for emphysema on diaphragm dimensions and configuration. Am J Respir Crit Care Med 2001;163(5):1171–5.

21. Fessler HE, Permutt S. Lung volume reduction surgery and airflow limitation. Am J Respir Crit Care Med 1998;157(3 Pt 1):715–22.

22. Cooper JD, Trulock EP, Triantafillou AN, et al. Bilateral pneumectomy (volume reduction) for chronic obstructive pulmonary disease. J Thorac Cardiovasc Surg 1995;109(1):106–9.

23. Wisser W, Tschernko EM, Wanke T, et al. Functional improvements in ventilatory mechanics after lung volume reduction surgery for homogeneous emphysema. Eur J Cardiothorac Surg 1997;12:525–30.

24. Hamacher J, Bloch KE, Stammberger U, et al. Two years' outcome of lung volume reduction surgery in different morphologic emphysema types. Ann Thorac Surg 1999;68(1792):1792–8.

25. Weder W, Tutic M, Lardinois D, et al. Persistent benefit from lung volume reduction surgery in patients with homogeneous emphysema. Ann Thorac Surg 2009; 87(1):229–36.

26. Slone RM, Gierada DS. Radiology of pulmonary emphysema and lung volume reduction surgery. Semin Thorac Cardiovasc Surg 1996;8(1):61–82.

27. Wisser W, Klepetko W, Kontrus M, et al. Morphologic grading of the emphysematous lung and its relation to improvement after lung volume reduction surgery. Ann Thorac Surg 1998;65(3):793–9.

28. McKenna RJ Jr, Brenner M, Fischel RJ, et al. Patient selection criteria for lung volume reduction surgery. J Thorac Cardiovasc Surg 1997;114(6):957–67.

29. Rogers RM, Coxson HO, Sciurba FC, et al. Preoperative severity of emphysema predictive of improvement after lung volume reduction surgery: use of CT morphometry. Chest 2000;118(5):1240–7.

30. Kotloff RM, Hansen-Flaschen J, Lipson DA, et al. Apical perfusion fraction as a predictor of short-term functional outcome following bilateral lung volume reduction surgery. Chest 2001;120:1609–15.

31. Weder W, Thurnheer R, Stammberger U, et al. Radiologic emphysema morphology is associated with outcome after surgical lung volume reduction. Ann Thorac Surg 1997;64(2):313–20.

32. Russi EWBK, Weder W. Functional and morphological heterogeneity of emphysema and its implication for selection of patients for lung volume reduction surgery. Eur Respir J 1999;14:230–6.

33. Thurnheer R, Engel H, Weder W, et al. Role of lung perfusion scintigraphy in relation to chest CT and pulmonary function in the evaluation of candidates for lung volume reduction surgery. Am J Respir Crit Care Med 1999;159:301–10.

34. Bloch KE, Georgescu CL, Russi EW, et al. Gain and subsequent loss of lung function after lung volume reduction surgery in cases of severe emphysema with different morphologic patterns. J Thorac Cardiovasc Surg 2002;123(5):845–54.

35. Imfeld Keb S, Weder W, Russi EW. The BODE index after lung volume reduction surgery correlates with survival. Chest 2006;129(4):873–8.

36. NETT. Rationale and design of the National Emphysema Treatment Trial (NETT): a prospective randomized trial of lung volume reduction surgery. J Thorac Cardiovasc Surg 2001;158(3):518–28.

Lung Volume Reduction Surgery for Patients with Alpha-1 Antitrypsin Deficiency Emphysema

James M. Donahue, MD[a], Stephen D. Cassivi, MD, MSc, FRCSC[b,c],*

KEYWORDS

- Emphysema • Surgery • Alpha-1 antitrypsin deficiency
- Lung volume reduction surgery

Alpha-1 antitrypsin deficiency (A1AD) is a rare genetic disorder characterized clinically by early-onset emphysema and, more rarely, liver disease and vasculitis. Recent advances in understanding the genetic basis of this disorder have enabled a more detailed understanding of its epidemiology. Alpha-1 antitrypsin is a serine protease inhibitor whose major function is to counteract the proteolytic activity of neutrophil elastase and trypsin. In the lungs, enhanced elastase activity results in accelerated parenchymal destruction leading to emphysematous changes predominantly in the lung bases. Medical treatment for this disorder includes standard therapies for emphysema and so-called augmentation therapy, consisting of the infusion of purified pooled plasma alpha-1 antitrypsin. Surgical options include lung transplantation and lung volume reduction surgery (LVRS). Although survival rates for patients who have A1AD after transplantation may approximate those of patients who have chronic obstructive pulmonary disease (COPD), donor availability limits its applicability. As with patients who have severe COPD, LVRS has been attempted in patients who have A1AD. The results of these studies form the basis for this review.

INCIDENCE AND PATHOPHYSIOLOGY

A1AD was first described in 1963 by Laurell and Eriksson at Lund University, Sweden.[1] Since that time, extensive population-based and molecular genetic research has enhanced the understanding of the epidemiology of A1AD. The estimated prevalence of A1AD is approximately 1.9% among patients who have emphysema. Accordingly, in the United States, the number of people who have symptomatic emphysema resulting from A1AD is believed approximately 60,000.[2–4]

A1AD is inherited in an autosomal codominant fashion. Approximately 100 separate alleles have been identified in the serine protease inhibitor gene, SERPINA1 (formerly called P_1) on the long arm of chromosome 14 (14q32.1).[5] The most common mutation gives rise to the Z allele and is caused by a glutamate to lysine mutation at position 342. This results in quantitative and functional deficiencies in alpha-1 antitrypsin such that patients who are homozygous ZZ typically produce only 10% to 15% of normal amounts of the protease inhibitor. People of northern European or Saudi Arabian ancestry have the highest rate of this genetic variant. Studies directly measuring the frequency of the ZZ genotype estimate its prevalence in the United States to be 1 in 4455, or approximately 66,000 individuals.[6–8]

Alpha-1 antitrypsin, a serine protease inhibitor, inactivates proteolytic enzymes, primarily neutrophil elastase and trypsin. In addition, alpha-1 antitrypsin has been shown to have anti-inflammatory properties, such as regulating the expression of

[a] Division of General Thoracic Surgery, University of Maryland, 22 South Greene Street, N4E35, Baltimore, MD 21201, USA
[b] Division of General Thoracic Surgery, Mayo Clinic, 200 First Street S.W., Rochester, MN 55905, USA
[c] William J. von Liebig Transplant Center, Mayo Clinic, Rochester, MN 55905, USA
* Corresponding author. Division of General Thoracic Surgery, Mayo Clinic, 200 First Street S.W., Rochester, MN 55905.
E-mail address: cassivi.stephen@mayo.edu (S.D. Cassivi).

Thorac Surg Clin 19 (2009) 201–208
doi:10.1016/j.thorsurg.2009.02.002
1547-4127/09/$ – see front matter © 2009 Elsevier Inc. All rights reserved.

pro-inflammatory cytokines.[9–11] It is produced primarily in the liver and reaches the lungs by diffusion from the circulation, although there is some local production of alpha-1 antitrypsin by macrophages and bronchial epithelial cells in the lungs.[12,13] Deficiencies in alpha-1 antitrypsin lead to accelerated pulmonary parenchymal destruction mediated by unopposed proteolytic action of neutrophil elastase and trypsin.

PRESENTATION AND MEDICAL THERAPY

Patients who have emphysema caused by A1AD generally develop onset of symptoms in the fourth or fifth decade. Despite this relatively early age of presentation, distinguishing patients who have A1AD from those who have COPD can be challenging. Distribution of the emphysematous changes in patients who have A1AD is panacinar and typically disproportionately affects the lung bases (**Figs. 1** and **2**).[14] Patients who have A1AD may, however, also develop emphysematous changes in an apical distribution. A recent study by Parr and colleagues[15] reported that more than one third of patients who had A1AD had an apical predominance of disease. Furthermore, as detailed in the National Heart, Lung, and Blood Institute (NHLBI) registry of patients who have A1AD, symptoms and presentation are similar to those experienced by most patients who have COPD.[16] These areas of overlap with COPD may explain why patients who have A1AD can experience a delay in diagnosis of up to 7 years from the onset of symptoms and why only 1% to 5% of patients who have severe A1AD are believed

to be diagnosed accurately.[8,17–19] Although most patients who have A1AD develop emphysema, up to 20% do not.[6,15]

Cigarette smoking is particularly hazardous for patients who have A1AD. Beyond the nonspecific inflammatory reaction that it causes in the airway and lung parenchyma, cigarette smoke also is known to directly inactivate alpha-1 antitrypsin by oxidizing methionine residues to sulfoxyl groups. Avoidance of cigarette smoking, therefore, is critical to averting accelerated disease progression. Data from the NHLBI registry show that the annual rate of decline in the forced expiratory volume in 1 second (FEV_1) in patients who have A1AD was 109 mL/year for smokers whereas it was 67 mL/year for never smokers and 54 mL/year for exsmokers.[16]

Perhaps the most important reason for accurately diagnosing patients who have A1AD is the potential improvement derived from infusion of purified plasma alpha-1 antitrypsin. The goal of augmentation therapy is to maintain serum alpha-1 antitrypsin levels above 11 μmol/L. Levels below this value have been shown to be associated with the development of symptomatic emphysema.[20] Generally, infusions must be administered on a weekly basis to maximize effectiveness. Although proved safe, augmentation therapy is expensive, with costs approximating $50,000 per year.[21] In terms of efficacy, observational data from the NHLBI registry suggest an improvement in survival rates and decrease in the decrement in FEV_1, most notably for patients who have moderate airflow obstruction.[22] Benefits for patients who have severe or mild airflow

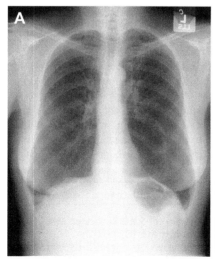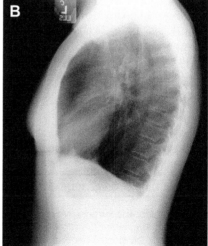

Fig. 1. Typical chest radiograph of a patient who had A1AD emphysema, demonstrating the hyperexpansion of the lungs, flattening of the domes of the diaphragm, and lower lung field predominance of the disease. (*A*) Posterior-anterior view; (*B*) lateral view.

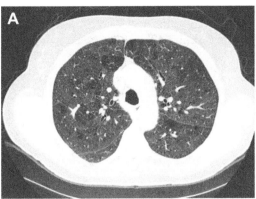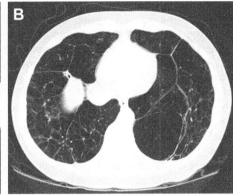

Fig. 2. Typical CT images of a patient who had A1AD emphysema, demonstrating predominance of disease in the lower lung fields. (*A*) Level of aortic arch showing some mild emphysematous changes; (*B*) level of lower lung fields just above the diaphragm demonstrating more severe emphysematous destruction of the lung parenchyma and resultant bullous type disease.

obstruction are less obvious. Once the FEV$_1$ is less than 35% predicted, augmentation therapy provides no measurable benefit. Given the expense and limited efficacy of augmentation therapy for patients who have A1AD and who have severe airflow obstruction, surgical options, including transplantation and LVRS, remain important therapeutic alternatives.

LUNG TRANSPLANTATION

According to the most recent International Society for Heart and Lung Transplantation registry data, 8% of lung transplants are performed for A1AD.[23] The Washington University experience of lung transplantation for A1AD by Cassivi and coworkers from 1988 to 2000 included 86 patients.[24] During that time period, 220 patients underwent transplantation for COPD. The patients who had A1AD were significantly younger, with a mean age of 49 compared, with patients who had COPD, whose mean age was 55. In this series bilateral lung transplantation was performed more frequently for A1AD (84.9%) than for COPD (66.8%). The 5-year survival rate for patients who had A1AD was 60.5%, which was not statistically different from the 56.8% 5-year survival rate for those who had COPD, despite the fact that, on average, the patients who had A1AD were a younger group.

Conversely, a recent review of the University of Toronto experience by de Perrot and colleagues from 1983 to 2003 showed worse survival for patients who had A1AD compared with those who had COPD.[25] During this time period, 88 transplants were performed for COPD, whereas 63 were performed for A1AD. Bilateral lung transplantation was performed for 83% of patients

who had emphysema with no report of differences between those who had COPD and those who had A1AD. After bilateral transplantation, 10-year survival rate for patients with COPD was 43% versus 23% for patients who had A1AD. This difference seemed to be due to the increased incidence in death from sepsis in patients who had A1AD relative to those who had COPD (27% versus 6%). The increased incidence of septic complications in patients who had A1AD may be related to deficiencies in antiprotease activity causing a blunted response to reperfusion injury and infection.[26] Whether or not a benefit exists in providing augmentation therapy post transplantation, particularly during periods of respiratory infection, is not known.[27]

LUNG VOLUME REDUCTION SURGERY

By removing the most diseased portions of the emphysematous lung, LVRS aims to improve the elastic recoil and provide more space for the otherwise compressed and comparatively less diseased remaining lung. Decreasing the amount of air space distention may help restore the diaphragm and other muscles of inspiration to more physiologic and ergonomic positions. This postulated improvement in respiratory mechanics and expiratory airflow is believed to result in less dyspnea. Early experience by Brantigan and colleagues, at the University of Maryland, showed that 75% of patients undergoing unilateral LVRS reported symptomatic improvement, although criteria for improvement were not clearly defined.[28] The operative mortality of 18% in the investigators' first cohort was a major factor in dampening enthusiasm for this new approach.

Renewed interest in LVRS for the treatment of severe emphysema was stimulated by the work of Cooper and coworkers at Washington University in the 1990s. Their report of 150 selected patients undergoing bilateral LVRS showed a 51% increase in FEV$_1$ and a 28% decrease in residual volume (RV) at 6 months.[29] Perioperative mortality was 4%. In addition, dyspnea scores improved significantly. Extended follow-up of these patients to 5 years by Ciccone and colleagues[30] revealed that the magnitude of the improvements in FEV$_1$ and RV diminished, although they remained significantly improved with respect to preoperative values. In the original series, 18 patients had lower lobe–predominant disease, 11 of whom had A1AD. Although improvements in FEV$_1$ and RV were seen in patients who have lower lobe–predominant disease at 6 months, they were significantly less than those seen in patients who had upper lobe–predominant disease.

The efficacy of LVRS has been examined in many randomized trials. The largest was the National Emphysema Treatment Trial (NETT), which randomized 1218 patients who had severe emphysema to LVRS or medical therapy. The results of this trial were reported in 2003 with follow-up for 2 years.[31] Although overall mortality between the LVRS and medically treated groups was similar, LVRS was associated with durable improvements in exercise capacity, lung function, and quality of life.

LVRS typically is performed via a median sternotomy or bilateral video-assisted thoracic surgical (VATS) approach. A nonrandomized comparison between these approaches in the NETT trial demonstrated no significant difference in terms of morbidity, mortality, or functional results. The VATS approach was associated with decreased hospital costs and earlier recovery.[32] Regardless of the approach, the procedure entails stapled resection of 20% to 30% of the volume of each lung. The diseased lung is removed with a continuous staple line reinforced with bovine pericardial strips to reduce air leaks (**Fig. 3**). Some diseased lung generally is left behind to avoid creating large air spaces that may predispose to persistent air leaks. If possible, patients should be extubated immediately after the procedure is completed. Chest tubes are left to water seal unless there is evidence of a large air space on CXR or a major air leak. Aggressive postoperative respiratory care, including liberal use of bronchoscopy to clear secretions, is imperative. With these maneuvers, length of stay after LVRS approximates 7 to 10 days with morbidity rates of 20% to 30%,

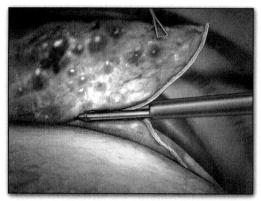

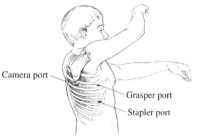

Camera port

Grasper port

Stapler port

Fig. 3. Illustration of thoracoscopic view of lower lobe LVRS in a patient who had A1AD emphysema with lower lobe–predominant disease. Volume reduction is done using an endoscopic stapling device and a buttressed staple line. (*Inset*) Lateral decubitus position and placement of port site incisions for thoracoscopic volume reduction.

primarily related to prolonged air leak and pneumonia.[29,30]

Although patients who have A1AD may have a variable distribution of diseased lung parenchyma, typically these patients have a predominance of disease in the lower segments of the lung. This is in contradistinction to the more common incidence of patients who have COPD resulting from cigarette smoking who typically have upper lobe–predominant disease when they have a heterogeneous distribution of disease. The different distribution of diseased lung in patients who have A1AD, therefore, requires a varied approach, where the more diseased lower segments are targeted for resection, rather than the more conventional upper lobe volume reduction that is commonly described.

There are limited data available for review on the application of LVRS to patients who have A1AD. Of the 1218 patients randomized in the NETT trial, only 1.3% had severe A1AD.[33] Eleven patients who had A1AD underwent LVRS in Cooper and colleagues' series (described previously) and five patients who had A1AD underwent LVRS in a series reported by Naunheim and associates at St. Louis University.[29,34] Specific follow-up of the patients who had A1AD were not available in these series. To date, follow-up of 66 patients who had A1AD and were undergoing LVRS have been reported. The relevant five series are listed in **Table 1**. In general, these series show marked improvements in dyspnea, 6-minute walk distances, and lung function testing during the first 6 to 12 months after LVRS. These parameters return to baseline within the next 1 to 2 years and then begin to decline. In series with follow-up greater than 1 year, however, patients continued to report less dyspnea. Most series include a group of patients who had COPD who underwent LVRS during the same time period. The patients who have COPD enjoy more sustained symptomatic and functional improvement. Despite the small number of patients, these studies are marked by differences in patient selection, distribution of emphysema, and surgical technique (see **Table 1**). There are no reports of perioperative mortality in these series, and morbidity rates approximate 30%, related primarily to pneumonia and prolonged air leak.

The first reported series was from Cassina and colleagues[35] in Germany. They reported on 12 patients, mean age 49 and mean preoperative FEV$_1$ of 24% of predicted. Five patients were former smokers. All patients were receiving monthly augmentation therapy for at least 2 years preoperatively, and this was continued post-operatively. In this study, LVRS was performed via bilateral muscle-sparing anteroaxillary thoracotomies. At 6 months, the dyspnea score decreased from 3.2 to 1.9 and FEV$_1$ increased to 34% of predicted. There also were decreases in RV and total lung capacity (TLC). By 1 year, these values returned to baseline and demonstrated continued deterioration by 2 years.

More encouraging results were reported by Gelb and colleagues,[36] who reviewed 6 patients who had a mean age of 61. Four patients were former smokers and mean preoperative FEV$_1$ in the four patients who have greater than 6-month follow-up was 30% of predicted. LVRS was confined to the lower lobes in these patients and was performed via a bilateral VATS approach. At a mean follow-up of 27 months, there was a small improvement in FEV$_1$ to 33% of predicted. Static lung volumes remained reduced and the dyspnea score had decreased from 3.2 to 2.2. In addition, static lung elastic recoil had improved.

The largest available series comes from Tutic and colleagues[37] in Switzerland. They prospectively followed 21 patients who had a median age of 56. The distribution of emphysematous changes in these patients was predominantly in the lower lobes in 10 patients, in the upper lobes in four, in both lobes in four, and homogenous in three. Fifteen patients had evidence of inflammatory changes on CT scan. Mean preoperative FEV$_1$ was 27% of predicted in the study cohort, 19 of whom were former smokers. These patients were quite symptomatic, with a preoperative dyspnea score of 3.7. LVRS was performed via a bilateral VATS approach. By 1 year, FEV$_1$ improved to 34% of predicted and the RV/TLC ratio had decreased from 67% to 54%. Six-minute walk distance increased from 278 m to 406 m and the dyspnea score decreased to 1.7. At 3 years, at which time 10 patients were available for evaluation, these values started to return to baseline, although the mean dyspnea score of 2.57 remained improved from baseline. The four patients who derived the longest-lasting benefit had heterogeneous emphysema and no

Table 1
Demographics of patients undergoing lung volume reduction surgery for alpha-1 antitrypsin deficiency emphysema

Author	n	Age	Distribution of Emphysema	Operative Approach
Cassina	12	49 (mean)	N/A	Bilateral anteroaxillary thoracotomy
Gelb	6	61 (mean)	Lower lobes—6	Bilateral VATS
Tutic	21	56 (median)	Lower lobes—10 Upper lobes—4 Both lobes—4 Homogenous—3	Bilateral VATS
Stoller	10	66 (median)	Lower lobes—3 Upper lobes—7	Bilateral VATS or median sternotomy
Dauriat	17	56 (mean)	Lower lobes—17	Unilateral thoracotomy

inflammatory changes on CT. Two of these patients had upper lobe–predominant disease. Twelve patients were eligible for transplantation at the time of LVRS. Six of these patients demonstrated symptomatic improvement whereas six subsequently underwent successful lung transplantation.

Stoller and colleagues[33] reported on 10 patients who had A1AD and who underwent LVRS as part of the NETT trial. Median age of these patients was 65.8 years. Mean preoperative FEV_1 was 27% of predicted and seven patients had upper lobe–predominant disease. Mean FEV_1 improved to 30% of predicted at 6 months but returned to 27.5% of predicted by 2 years. RV decreased by 43.5% at 6 months and was still decreased by 36.5% at 2 years. St. George's Respiratory Questionnaire scores increased by 4.6 at 6 months but had decreased by 4.4 at 2 years. When compared with six patients who had severe A1AD and who were randomized to medical therapy, 2-year mortality was 20% for the LVRS group and none for those treated medically. As reported by the investigators, 2-year mortality for alpha-1 antitrypsin–replete patients in the NETT trial was 17.6%. None of the 10 patients who had A1AD and who underwent LVRS were in the upper lobe–predominant, low-exercise capacity group who derived the maximum benefit from LVRS in the NETT trial.

Dauriat and colleagues[38] in France reported on 17 patients who had a mean age of 56 years. Preoperatively, 16 of the patients required supplemental oxygen at rest. LVRS was confined to the lower lobes in these patients and was performed via a unilateral thoracotomy. Mean preoperative FEV_1 was 22% of predicted and improved to 29% of predicted by 3 to 6 months. By 1 year, it had decreased to 26% of predicted but was still significantly improved from baseline. Mean dyspnea score had improved from 4.2 to 3.1 at 3 to 6 months after LVRS and remained significantly improved from baseline at 3.2 at 1 year after surgery. Six-minute walk distance increased from 237 m to 310 m at 3 to 6 months but declined to 270 m at 1 year. Total lung capacity decreased moderately from 138% of predicted preoperatively to 132% of predicted at 3 to 6 months and 133% at 1 year after surgery.

Given the scarcity of donors for lung transplantation, LVRS has been used as a bridge for patients who have severe emphysema and who are eligible for transplantation. Uncertainty exists as to the likelihood of subsequently requiring a transplant and on the outcome of transplantation in this setting. The use of this strategy for patients who have A1AD has been limited. As described previously, of the 12 patients eligible for transplant at the time of LVRS in Tutic and coworkers' study, six later underwent successful transplantation whereas the other six remained improved symptomatically.[37] In a report from Washington University, Meyers and colleagues[39] describe the outcome of 99 patients who were eligible for transplantation but underwent LVRS. In this series, there were four perioperative and 17 late deaths. Thirty-two of the remaining 78 patients were listed for transplantation. Fifteen patients eventually received a transplant at a mean interval of 3.8 years from the time of LVRS. All patients survived the transplant operation. Three patients died later from rejection or infection. In this series, 10 patients had A1AD. Six of these patients subsequently required transplant and two died before being listed. Zenati and colleagues[40] from the University of Pittsburgh reported on 20 transplant-eligible patients who had emphysema and who underwent LVRS. Two of these patients had A1AD, although the specific outcomes of these patients were not reported. Overall, at a mean follow-up of 32 months, there was one late death, one patient underwent successful transplantation, two were listed for transplant, and 15 remained off the transplant list. A single report exists from the University of Toronto program where a woman who had A1AD underwent simultaneous right single lung transplant and left LVRS via a clamshell incision. In this case report, initial postoperative function was improved but no long-term follow-up was reported.[41]

SUMMARY

Currently, A1AD is recognized in approximately 2% of patients who have emphysema, although this may be an underestimation of the prevalence of this disease. Given the relatively young age at which patients who have A1AD present with emphysema, therapies aimed at slowing the progression of this disease are imperative. In addition to abstaining from smoking, the use of augmentation therapy may benefit some patients who have moderate airflow obstruction. For patients who have severe airflow obstruction, the most effective therapy is surgical. Despite a possible increased risk for infectious complications, transplantation remains a viable option for these patients who have long-term results mirroring those of patients transplanted for smoking-related COPD. Given limited donor availability, however, LVRS must be considered in these patients possibly as definitive therapy but more likely as a bridge to transplantation. LVRS for patients who have A1AD remains relatively uncommon despite a general perception that it remains a surgical option. In a survey of European thoracic surgical centers, Hamacher and colleagues[42] found that two thirds of respondents included A1AD in their list of indications for LVRS. Although the durability of the benefits derived from LVRS in patients who have A1AD seems inferior to that of patients who have COPD, the available data show improved 6-minute walk distances and decreased dyspnea persisting for 1 to 2 years after LVRS in patients who had A1AD. Further experience is necessary to determine whether or not subgroups of patients who have A1AD, such as those who have clear heterogeneous distribution, may derive more long-lasting improvement from LVRS.

REFERENCES

1. Laurell C-B, Eriksson A. The electrophoretic alpha 1-globulin pattern of serum in alpha 1-antitrypsin deficiency. Scand J Clin Lab Invest 1963;15:132–40.
2. Stoller JK, Aboussouan LS. Alpha 1-antitrypson deficiency. Lancet 2005;365:2225–36.
3. Lethbridge-Cejku M, Schiller JS, Bernadel L. Vital and Health Statistics, series 10, number 222: summary health statistics for US adults-National Health Interview Survey, 2002. Hyattsville (MD): National Center for Health Statistics, 2004. Available at: http://ww.cdc.gov/nchs/data/series/sr_10/sr10_222.pdf. Accessed April 18, 2008.
4. Lieberman J, Winter B, Sastre A. Alpha 1-antitrypsin Pi-types in 965 COPD patients. Chest 1986;89:370–3.
5. DeMeo DL, Silverman EK. Alpha 1-antitrypsin deficiency, 2:genetic aspects of alpha(1)-antitrypsin deficiency: phenotypes and genetic modifiers of emphysema risk. Thorax 2004;59:259–64.
6. Eriksson S. A 30-year perspective on alpha 1-antitrypsin deficiency. Chest 1996;110(Suppl 6):237S–42S.
7. Gadek JE, Crystal RG. Alpha 1-antitrypsin deficiency. In: Stanbury JB, Wyngaarden JB, Frederickson DS, et al, editors. The metabolic basis of inherited disease. New York: McGraw-Hill; 1983. p. 1450–67.
8. Tobin MJ, Cook PJ, Hutchison DC. Alpha 1 antitrypsin deficiency: the clinical and physiological features of pulmonary emphysema in subjects homozygous for Pi type Z—a survey by the British Thoracic Association. Br J Dis Chest 1983;77:14–27.
9. Stockley RA, Bayley DL, Unsal I, et al. The effect of augmentation therapy on bronchial inflammation in alpha 1-antitrypsin deficiency. Am J Respir Crit Care Med 2002;165:1494–8.
10. Aldonyte R, Jansson L, Janciauskiene S. Concentration-dependent effects of native and polymerized alpha 1-antityrpsin on primary human monocytes, in vitro. BMC Cell Biol 2004;5:11.
11. Janciauskiene S, Larsson S, Larsson P, et al. Inhibition of lipopolysaccharide-mediated human monocyte activation, in vitro, by alpha 1-antitrypsin. Biochem Biophys Res Commun 2004;321:592–600.
12. Lomas DA, Mahadeva R. Alpha 1-antitrypsin polymerization and the serpinopathies: pathobiology and prospects for therapy. J Clin Invest 2002;110:1585–90.
13. Stecenko A, Brigham KL. Gene therapy progress and prospects: alpha-1 antitrypsin. Gene Ther 2003;10:95–9.
14. Stavngaard T, Shaker SB, Dirksen A. Quantitative assessment of emphysema distribution in smokers and patients with alpha1-antitrypsin deficiency. Respir Med 2006;100(1):94–100.
15. Parr DG, Stoel BC, Stolk J, et al. Pattern of emphysema distribution in alpha 1-antitrypsin deficiency influences lung function impairment. Am J Respir Crit Care Med 2004;170(11):1172–8.
16. McElvaney NG, Stoller JK, Buist AS, et al. Baseline characteristics of enrollees in the national heart, lung and blood institute registry of α_1-antitrypsin deficiency. Chest 1997;111:394–403.
17. Stoller JK, Smith P, Yang P, et al. Physical and social impact of alpha-1 antitrypsin deficiency: results of a survey. Cleve Clin J Med 1994;61:461–7.
18. Silverman EK, Miletich JP, Pierce JA, et al. Alpha 1-antitrypsin deficiency: high prevalence in the St. Louis area determined by direct population screening. Am Rev Respir Dis 1989;140:961–6.
19. Luisetti M, Seersholm N. Alpha 1-antitripsin deficiency, 1: epidemiology of alpha 1-antitrypsin deficiency. Thorax 2004;59:164–9.
20. American Thoracic Society/European Respiratory Society statement: standards for the diagnosis and management of individuals with alpha-1 antitrypsin deficiency. Am J Respir Crit Care Med 2003;168:818–900.
21. The Alpha-1 antitrypsin Deficiency Registry Study Group. A registry of patients with severe deficiency of alpha 1-antitrypsin: design and methods. Chest 1994;106:1223–32.
22. Alpha 1-Antitrypsin Deficiency Registry Study Group. Survival and FEV1 decline in individuals with severe deficiency of alpha1-antitrypsin. Am J Respir Crit Care Med 1998;158:49–59.
23. Trulock EP, Christie JD, Edwards LB, et al. Registry of the International Society for Heart and Lunch Transplantation: twenty-fourth Official Adult Lung and Heart-Lung Transplantation Report-2007. J Heart Lung Transplant 2007;26:782–95.

24. Cassivi SD, Meyers BF, Battafarano RJ, et al. Thirteen-year experience in lung transplantation for emphysema. Ann Thorac Surg 2002;74:1663–70.

25. de Perrot M, Chaparro C, McRae K, et al. Twenty-year experience of lung transplantation at a single center: influence of recipient diagnosis on long-term survival. J Thorac Cardiovasc Surg 2004;127:1493–501.

26. Meyer KC, Nunley DR, Dauber JH, et al. Neutrophils, unopposed neutrophil elastase and alpha 1-antiprotease defenses following human lung transplantation. Am J Respir Crit Care Med 2001;164:97–102.

27. Trulock EP. Lung transplantation for α_1-antitrypsin deficiency emphysema. Chest 1996;110:284S–94S.

28. Brantigan OC, Mueller E, Kress MB. A surgical approach to pulmonary emphysema. Am Rev Respir Dis 1959;80:194–206.

29. Cooper JD, Patterson GA, Sundaresan RS, et al. Results of 150 consecutive bilateral lung volume reduction procedures in patients with severe emphysema. J Thorac Cardiovasc Surg 1996;112:1319–30.

30. Ciccone AM, Meyers BF, Guthrie TJ, et al. Long-term outcome of bilateral lung volume reduction in 250 consecutive patients with emphysema. J Thorac Cardiovasc Surg 2003;125:513–25.

31. Fishman F, Martinez F, Naunheim K, et al. A randomized trial comparing lung-volume-reduction surgery with medical therapy for severe emphysema. N Engl J Med 2003;348:2059–73.

32. McKenna RJ, Benfitt JO, DeCamp M, et al. Safety and efficacy of median sternotomy versus video-assisted thoracic surgery for lung volume reduction surgery. J Thorac Cardiovasc Surg 2004;127(5):1350–60.

33. Stoller JK, Gildea TR, Ries AL, et al. Lung volume reduction surgery in patients with emphysema and α-1 antitrypsin deficiency. Ann Thorac Surg 2007;83:241–51.

34. Naunheim KS, Keller CA, Krucylak PE, et al. Unilateral video-assisted thoracic surgical lung reduction. Ann Thorac Surg 1996;61:1092–8.

35. Cassina PC, Teschler H, Konietzko N, et al. Two-year results after lung reduction volume reduction surgery in α_1-antitrypsin deficiency versus smokers emphysema. Eur Respir J 1998;12:1028–32.

36. Gelb AF, McKenna RJ, Brenner M, et al. Lung reduction after bilateral lower lobe lung volume reduction surgery for α_1-antitrypsin emphysema. Eur Respir J 1999;14:928–33.

37. Tutic M, Bloch KE, Lardinois D, et al. Long-term results after lung volume reduction surgery in patients with α_1-antitrypsin deficiency. J Thorac Cardiovasc Surg 2004;128:408–13.

38. Dauriat G, Mal H, Jebrak G, et al. Functional results of unilateral lung volume reduction surgery in alpha1-antitrypsin deficient patients. Int J Chron Obstruct Pulmon Dis 2006;1(2):201–6.

39. Meyers BF, Yusen RD, Guthrie TJ, et al. Outcome of bilateral lung volume reduction in patients with emphysema potentially eligible for lung transplantation. J Thorac Cardiovasc Surg 2001;122:10–7.

40. Zenati M, Keenan RJ, Courcoulas AP, et al. Lung volume reduction or lung transplantation for end-state pulmonary emphysema. Eur J Cardiothorac Surg 1998;14:27–32.

41. Todd TR, Perron J, Winton TL, et al. Simultaneous single-lung transplantation and lung volume reduction. Ann Thorac Surg 1997;63(5):1468–70.

42. Hamacher J, Russi EW, Weder W. Lung volume reduction surgery: a survey on the European experience. Chest 2000;117(6):1560–7.

Concomitant Lung Cancer Resection and Lung Volume Reduction Surgery

Cliff K. Choong, MBBS, FRACS, FRCS[a,b,c,*],
Balakrishnan Mahesh, MBBS, MD[a],
G. Alexander Patterson, MD[d], Joel D. Cooper, MD[e]

KEYWORDS

- Lung volume reduction surgery • Emphysema
- Wedge resection • Lobectomy • Lung cancer

Early-stage non–small cell lung cancer is best treated by complete anatomic resection. Patients who have resectable lung cancer but associated advanced emphysema are often precluded from surgery because of severe respiratory limitation. For these patients, alternative treatment strategies, including radiation therapy with or without chemotherapy, are considered less than optimal and yield comparatively poor results. Furthermore, conventional radiation therapy may lead to the same degree of reduction in pulmonary function as surgical resection. Stereotactic body radiation therapy has been proposed as an alternative local treatment option for high-risk patients who have early-stage lung cancer and is undergoing evaluation. Patients who have severely limited pulmonary function represent a management problem for the radiation oncologist and for the surgeon. This dilemma is further compounded for surgeons by the lack of a precisely definable point at which the risk-to-benefit ratio for resection becomes unfavorable, particularly in light of improvements in the anesthetic, surgical, and postoperative treatment of patients who have advanced emphysema.

Certain highly selected patients who have clinically resectable lung cancer and severe respiratory limitation due to emphysema may have an acceptable operative risk and functional improvements by combining a suitable cancer resection with lung volume reduction surgery (LVRS).[1–20] This combination would provide the best treatment of early-stage lung cancer while being a palliative treatment of the symptoms of emphysema. Several groups have evaluated their experience of combined lung cancer resection and LVRS and have reported beneficial early and long-term results.[1–20] This article provides a review in this area and recommends surgical strategies in this group of patients who have concomitant lung cancer and severe emphysema.

PATIENT EVALUATION AND SELECTION

Most groups follow a specific institutional protocol in the patient evaluation and selection process for concomitant surgery.[1,7,9,12,13] These are not too dissimilar among the different groups, however. Assessment for the suitability of LVRS

C.K.C and B.M. are equal first co-authors on this article.
a Papworth Hospital NHS Foundation Trust, Cambridge, UK
b Department of Surgery, The University of Cambridge, Cambridge, UK
c Monash University, Monash Medical Centre, 246 Clayton Road, Clayton, Victoria 3168, Australia
d Division of Cardiothoracic Surgery, Washington University School of Medicine, Barnes-Jewish Hospital, St. Louis, MO, USA
e Division of Thoracic Surgery, Hospital of the University of Pennsylvania, Philadelphia, PA, USA
* Corresponding author. Department of Surgery (MMC), Monash University, Block E, Level 5, Monash Medical Centre, 246 Clayton Road, Clayton, Victoria 3168, Australia.
E-mail address: cliffchoong@hotmail.com (C.K. Choong).

Thorac Surg Clin 19 (2009) 209–216
doi:10.1016/j.thorsurg.2009.04.004
1547-4127/09/$ – see front matter © 2009 Elsevier Inc. All rights reserved.

includes history, physical examination, pulmonary function tests with lung volumes, arterial blood gas analysis (at rest on room air), chest radiograph, standardized CT of the chest, radionuclide ventilation-perfusion lung scan, 6-minute walk test, and dyspnea scale, such as the Medical Research Council dyspnea scale or other types. Systemic spread of lung cancer disease was additionally evaluated by CT of the abdomen and pelvis, brain CT, and positron emission tomography–CT scan. Details of the selection process for lung volume reduction have been reported.[21–28] Marked hyperinflation of the chest and adequate regional distinction in the destruction pattern of emphysema to provide target areas of useless lung accessible to surgical resection were critical selection criteria in all patients.[21–28] Patients who are offered concomitant surgery are highly selected and must fulfill the criteria set out for both LVRS and cancer surgery.[29,30]

Various methods have been reported to determine suitability for pulmonary resection in patients who have moderate to severe respiratory limitation.[1,3–6,9,12,19] Korst and colleagues[4] noted an improvement or minimal loss of pulmonary function following lobectomy for the treatment of non–small cell lung carcinoma in 13 patients who had a forced expiratory volume in 1 second (FEV_1) of less than or equal to 60% of predicted value and an FEV_1/forced vital capacity (FVC) ratio of less than or equal to 0.6. They used a chronic obstructive pulmonary disease (COPD) index, a scoring system combining these two parameters, which helped to identify patients who may have only a limited reduction or even an improvement of pulmonary function following lobectomy. Carretta and coworkers[5] reported a subgroup of 10 patients in whom a higher radiologic visual assessment of emphysema severity in the affected lobe correlated to an unchanged or even an increase of pulmonary function following a lobectomy. The radiologic visual assessment used a scoring system that is a sum of the grading score of emphysema seen on chest radiograph and chest CT scan. Edwards and colleagues[6] extended the selection criteria for lobectomy to patients who had a predicted postoperative FEV_1 of less than 40% if the tumor was resectable, in whom the target lobe was both emphysematous and contributed to less than 10% of overall perfusion, and who had evidence of hyperinflation on radiologic assessment. Despite these various reported methods, no single test has been found to best define the patients who will and will not tolerate resection. Instead, these investigations, together with the physical condition of the patient

and the surgeon's experience, help to select patients suitable for combined surgical resection.

The patients judged suitable for surgery are enrolled in a preoperative pulmonary rehabilitation and smoking cessation program lasting 6 to 8 weeks. Patients are then reassessed the week before surgery by an interval history, physical examination, and investigations. In selected patients who are assessed to be in suitable physical condition at the time of initial evaluation, surgery may be considered without additional pulmonary rehabilitation. Patients who are offered concomitant surgery are highly selected and must satisfy the strict criteria set out for both LVRS and cancer surgery.

INTRAOPERATIVE SURGICAL STRATEGIES

Various intraoperative strategies have been used to perform the combined surgery. The decision to perform either a wedge resection or a lobectomy depends on the size and location of the tumor and the distribution and severity of the emphysema. Lobectomy is generally not performed in patients who have severe emphysema unless there is a heterogenous distribution of emphysema and the tumor is located within a destroyed, virtually functionless lobe. If the tumor is in the middle lobe and there are suitable target areas for LVRS in other lobes, then a middle lobectomy may be performed in conjunction with ipsilateral or bilateral LVRS. If the tumor is located in the best-preserved lobe other than the middle lobe, then either a wedge resection is performed or the patient is considered not to be a suitable candidate. An ipsilateral or contralateral LVRS is added to the cancer resection if there is a suitable target area for LVRS such that the resection would be expected to result in a likely improvement in the patient's postoperative pulmonary function. The type of combined surgery therefore depends on the location of the lung cancer and the distribution and severity of the emphysema. These strategies are combined with the standard systematic lymph node staging for lung cancer.

A flexible bronchoscopy with bronchial washings for gram stain and culture is performed at the beginning of the procedure, which helps to guide postoperative antibiotic management if the patient develops postoperative chest infection. If thick sticky mucus is encountered during bronchoscopy, this should be suctioned out. The presence of sticky mucus alerts the surgical team and lowers the threshold for consideration of flexible bronchoscopy or mini-tracheostomy for suctioning of secretions during the postoperative period.

The intraoperative strategies for a concomitant cancer resection and lung volume reduction surgery include:

1. Lobectomy only.[1–9,12–14] This procedure is usually performed in the setting of an upper-lobe lung cancer in a patient who has upper lobe–predominant severe emphysema in which the lobe has been severely destroyed by the emphysematous process and is virtually functionless. A lobectomy in such instance serves to treat both diseases well.[1–9,12–14] Rarely, a lower lobectomy is performed in a patient who has a lower-lobe lung cancer who also has lower lobe–predominant emphysema.[1] It is rare, however, to have lower lobe–predominant severe emphysema because the smoking-related emphysematous process usually predominantly affects both the upper lobes.

2. Lobectomy and contralateral LVRS.[1] This procedure is performed in the setting of an upper-lobe lung cancer in patients who have bilateral upper lobe–predominant severe emphysema. A median sternotomy can be used because this surgical approach provides access to both lungs through a single incision. An upper lobectomy in combination with a contralateral LVRS is then performed. Sequential bilateral video-assisted thoracoscopic surgery (VATS) or sequential thoracotomies in the same surgical setting are alternative surgical approaches when a median sternotomy is not the surgeon's preferred surgical approach or considered not to be the optimal approach. Apart from upper lobectomy, middle or lower lobectomy in combination with contralateral LVRS can also be undertaken and has been reported previously.[1] The decision to perform either an upper lobectomy alone or lobectomy in combination with contralateral LVRS depends on the distribution and severity of the emphysematous disease and the surgeon's personal experience and preference.

3. Ipsilateral middle lobectomy and LVRS.[1] This procedure is used in patients who have a right middle-lobe lung cancer with upper lobe–predominant emphysema. The middle lobectomy in combination with ipsilateral upper-lobe LVRS in such patients allows for treatment of both diseases through a right-sided surgical approach.[1]

4. Unilateral LVRS. This strategy is useful and simple for the treatment of an upper-lobe lung cancer that is situated within the resection target area of an upper-lobe LVRS. A large wedge resection of the upper lobe serves to remove both the lung cancer and a significant part of the upper lobe emphysematous disease. This operation is simple and relatively quick to perform. It has the disadvantage, however, that only a wedge resection is performed for the lung cancer, whereas lobectomy is considered a better oncologic operation and is currently the gold standard in the treatment of lung cancer. The decision to perform either an upper lobectomy or just a large upper-lobe wedge resection would depend on the size of the tumor, the location of the tumor, and the distribution of the upper-lobe emphysematous disease. A large tumor or a tumor situated outside the usual resection area of an upper-lobe LVRS may not be amendable to a large wedge resection and would be better treated by a lobectomy. An upper lobe that is virtually destroyed and functionless would also be served by a lobectomy rather than a large wedge resection.[1,7]

5. Ipsilateral lower-lobe wedge resection and upper-lobe LVRS.[1] When the cancer is located in a well-preserved lower lobe in a patient who has an upper lobe–predominant emphysema, a wedge resection of the lower-lobe lung cancer in combination with an ipsilateral upper-lobe LVRS can be performed.[1]

6. Bilateral LVRS.[1] This procedure is particularly suitable in patients who have a small upper-lobe lung cancer that is situated within the target resection area for LVRS. A bilateral LVRS in such a case would remove the upper lobe lung cancer and also palliate the emphysematous diseases on both lungs. A less aggressive approach in the management of the emphysema can be considered and adopted by performing a unilateral LVRS.[23]

7. Wedge resection and contralateral LVRS.[1] This procedure is rarely performed and is in the setting of a lower-lobe lung cancer in patients who have predominant contralateral upper-lobe severe emphysema. It may also be used for a small apical upper-lobe tumor with bilateral upper-lobe emphysema. A median sternotomy may provide adequate access to both lungs and allows for wedge resection of a peripheral lower-lobe lung cancer and contralateral LVRS. Alternatively, a bilateral sequential VATS or thoracotomy approach can be used if a median sternotomy approach is deemed to be less optimal. The scenario of predominant contralateral upper-lobe emphysema is generally rare because the emphysematous disease from smoking-related causes is generally a bilateral process.

It can thus be seen that there are several potential options in dealing with a patient who has a concomitant lung cancer and severe emphysema. The choice of technique applied depends on the location and size of the tumor, the severity and distribution of the emphysema, and the surgeon's experience and preference.

POSTOPERATIVE MANAGEMENT

Immediate extubation in the operating room or shortly thereafter in the postanesthesia recovery area is desirable and can generally be achieved.[1,6,21] During the postoperative period, patients are managed in a specialized thoracic step-down unit providing specialized postoperative nursing care. Optimal pain management is of utmost importance and generally a thoracic epidural catheter for continuous analgesia is placed before surgery and is used during the procedure and the postoperative period. It decreases the need for systemic narcotics and provides optimal pain management with minimal risk for respiratory depression. Most institutions have an acute pain service team with their preferred postoperative analgesic regimens. It is important that the members of the pain team regularly review the patients and apply the analgesic regimen to ensure that the patients are comfortable and are free of postoperative pain. This monitoring allows the patients to comply with the breathing and exercise programs. Chest physiotherapy and ambulation are generally initiated early by experienced physical therapists and thoracic surgical nurses, and these are continued throughout the hospital stay. Postoperative bedside bronchoscopy and mini-tracheostomy placement to clear secretions are rarely required. They should be considered in patients who are unable to clear their secretions, however, particularly in the presence of thick secretions, mucus plugging, and complications, such as lobar collapse.

OUTCOMES AND DISCUSSIONS

Choong and colleagues[1] from St. Louis reported their experience with 21 patients who underwent combined surgery using various strategies. The patients had a mean preoperative FEV_1 of 0.7 ± 0.2 L (29% predicted), residual volume (RV) of 5.5 ± 1.0 L (271%), and diffusing capacity for carbon monoxide of 8.0 ± 2.2 mL/min/mm Hg (34% predicted). In 9 patients, the cancer was located in a severely emphysematous lobe and the lung volume reduction surgery component of the procedure was accomplished with lobectomy

alone. In the remaining 12 patients, the cancer resection (lobectomy in 9 and wedge resection in 3 patients) was supplemented with LVRS using various strategies. There was no hospital mortality. The final pathologic staging among the 21 patients was stage I in 16 patients, stage II in 2 patients, and stage III in 2 patients. One patient was found to have stage IV disease in the old TNM staging system because of multifocal tumors in separate lobes. The postoperative complications encountered included prolonged air leak in 11 patients, atrial fibrillation in 6 patients, and reintubation for ventilatory assistance in 2 patients. The survival was 100% and 62.7% at 1 and 5 years, respectively. The Kaplan-Meier estimation of freedom from cancer recurrence at 1, 3, and 5 years was 90.5%, 84.0%, and 68.7%, respectively. The Kaplan-Meier estimation of freedom from cancer recurrence in patients who had stage I disease at 1, 3, and 5 years was 90.0%, 84.0%, and 69.3%, respectively. All patients showed improved lung function postoperatively. There was significant improvement in the FEV_1 and RV between preoperative values and each time point of follow-up through 3 years. The mean preoperative FEV_1 was 29% predicted, and the postoperative FEV_1 was 40%, 43%, 34%, and 28% predicted at 6 months, 1, 3, and 5 years, respectively. The mean preoperative RV was 271%, and the postoperative RV was 152%, 161%, 163%, and 195% predicted at 6 months, 1, 3, and 5 years, respectively. Although the FEV_1 returned to baseline by 5 years, the RV remained significantly improved in the group of patients. As with LVRS patients in general, there was no significant difference between the initial evaluation and post-rehabilitation FEV_1 and RV measurements. The diffusing capacity for carbon monoxide remained unchanged throughout all time points. There was substantial decrease in supplemental oxygen requirements at rest after surgery (57% preoperatively versus 6%, 18%, and 20% at 1, 3, and 5 years after surgery, respectively). Before surgery, 86% of the patients required supplemental oxygen with exertion and this decreased significantly following surgery. At 1, 3, and 5 years the requirement was 47%, 55%, and 80%, respectively. The patients also had functional improvement as measured by the 6-minute walk test. There was significant improvement in preoperative physical stamina in those patients who underwent pulmonary rehabilitation highlighting the importance of pulmonary rehabilitation. Further improvement in performance was evident after surgery and this improvement was maintained throughout follow-up with a gradual decline toward baseline at 5 years. Most of the patients

(89%) reported improvement in symptoms of dyspnea at 6 months following surgery. At 1 year 88% remained improved, 8% were unchanged, and 4% showed worsening. These improvements were sustained throughout follow-up, with only 17% of patients measured reporting a worse score at 5 years than their preoperative level. The study by Choong and coauthors[1] provided comprehensive follow-up data on the outcome of successful combined surgery. In their series, all patients had preoperative pulmonary function values in one or more categories well below the traditionally accepted minimal criteria for lobectomy. Following the combined surgery, these patients reported early and long-term benefits similar to those who had LVRS alone.[21,22,31,32] These early improvements were followed by a slow gradual decline of the pulmonary function tests, similar to the patients who had LVRS alone. The Kaplan-Meier estimation of survival at 1, 3, and 5 years in this group of patients was 100%, 73.7%, and 62.7%, respectively, and compares well to the reported long-term outcome of bilateral lung volume reduction in 250 consecutive patients who had emphysema, whereas the Kaplan-Meier estimation of survival at 1, 3, and 5 years was 93.6%, 84.4%, and 67.7%, respectively.[21] Choong and colleagues[1] concluded that concomitant lung cancer resection and LVRS allows highly selected patients who have early lung cancer and advanced emphysema to undergo the optimal treatment modality of cancer resection at a low risk with improvement of their pulmonary status.

McKenna and coauthors reported on 11 patients who had lung cancer and emphysema who underwent cancer resection by wedge resection (n = 7) or by lobectomy (n = 4) along with bilateral LVRS. They reported only one death in the follow-up period, and good functional improvement in all but one patient whose tumor was located in the middle lobe, which was the best lung tissue.[3]

Several groups have reported on the outcomes of lobectomy for the management of lung cancer in patients who have severe emphysema.[1-9,12-14] Low hospital mortality and good early and long-term outcomes were achieved. Carretta and colleagues[5] reported on 10 patients who underwent lobectomy for cancer within an emphysematous lobe. The patients had an improvement in FEV₁, FVC, and a decrease in airway resistance, implying significant improvement in lung and airway mechanics. Edwards and colleagues[6] from Leicester reported their experience of performing lobectomy in 29 patients who had a resectable lung cancer located within a poorly perfused, hyperinflated emphysematous lobe identified by radionuclide perfusion scintigraphy and CT scanning. They divided patients into two groups and compared the perioperative changes in spirometric parameters between Group A, 14 patients who had a mean preoperative FEV_1 less than 40%, versus Group B, 15 patients who had a mean preoperative FEV_1 greater than 40%. The study found that following surgery, patients in group B had a significant perioperative reduction in FEV_1 but in group A the FEV_1 did not change significantly after lobectomy. The mean difference in perioperative change between groups A and B was 331 mL. Despite the difference in preoperative FEV_1 between the groups, there was no difference in actual FEV_1 at 3 months' follow-up. The in-hospital mortality was 14% in group A and 0% in group B, although at a median follow up of 12 months with a range of 6 to 40 months there was no difference in survival between the groups. The authors concluded that the selection for lung cancer resection in patients who have emphysema using standard calculations of preoperative FEV_1 may be misleading and the effect of lobar volume reduction allows for an extension of the selection criteria.

The group from Leicester conducted another study to compare the outcomes of upper lobectomy versus upper-lobe LVRS. Their aim was to determine whether the physiologic benefits of this approach were superior to conventional nonanatomic lung volume reduction surgery. The lobectomy group consisted of 34 consecutive patients who underwent upper lobectomy for completely resected stage I or II non–small cell lung cancer and who had severe heterogeneous emphysema of apical distribution with a predicted postoperative FEV_1 of less than 40%. The upper-lobe LVRS group consisted of 46 similar patients (who did not have lung cancer) who underwent unilateral upper-lobe LVRS during the same period. The study found that there was no significant difference in median survival. The lobectomy patients had a shorter air leak duration (5 days versus 9 days) and hospital stay (8 days versus 13 days). The authors concluded that lobectomy for lung cancer in patients who have severe heterogenous emphysema is associated with similar improvement as conventional LVRS, but is associated with a shorter postoperative course. Lobectomy may therefore offer a therapeutic alternative to conventional LVRS in a selected population.

In a study to identify criteria that will preoperatively identify a group of patients who will not lose further function after lobectomy, Korst and colleagues[4] evaluated their patient cohort who had a preoperative FEV_1 of less than 80%. Over a 2-year period, they identified 13 patients who underwent lobectomy and had minimal change or improvement in the ventilatory function during a follow-up period ranging from 4 months to 2 years. These patients had undergone lobectomy alone as a form of combined lung cancer resection and LVRS. There was a mean increase in FEV_1 of 3.7% and FEV_1/FVC of 12.6%. These patients were highly selected using a COPD index, which was formulated by the authors. The COPD index grades the severity and purity of emphysematous disease. It is calculated by adding the preoperative FEV_1 (% of predicted in decimal form) to the preoperative ratio of FEV_1/FVC. The patients who have the lowest COPD index are those who have the most pure and severe disease. For example, if a patient has an FEV_1 of 60% of predicted and the FEV_1/FVC ratio is 0.5, the COPD index would be 0.6 plus 0.5, or 1.1. The 13 patients had a preoperative FEV_1 of less than or equal to 60% of predicted combined with a preoperative FEV_1/FVC ratio less than or equal to 0.6. The study showed that as the preoperative COPD index falls below 1.0, implying more severe and pure obstructive disease, the more likely it is that FEV_1 will increase after lobectomy. The COPD index, as defined by Korst and colleagues,[4] is thus an attempt to identify those patients who have the most severe and pure emphysematous disease. When this index falls below 1.0, there is a high likelihood that either little change will occur in the FEV_1 after lobectomy or this volume will increase. Patients who have a low preoperative FEV_1 but a COPD index greater than 1.2 are likely to have a restrictive disease and can be expected to sustain a 5% to 20% loss of function (FEV_1) after lobectomy. It is extremely important that the COPD index is carefully correlated with the distribution and severity of emphysema as assessed by CT scan and ventilation-perfusion scan. Patients who have a COPD index of less than 1.0 and a heterogeneous pattern of COPD in which the relatively nonfunctioning lobe is not resected will lose a large percentage of their FEV_1 with resection of a functioning lobe. In this study, 1 patient lost 58.6% of his preoperative FEV_1 after a left upper lobectomy, despite a COPD index of only 1.03. A close examination of his preoperative ventilation-perfusion scan revealed that his remaining left lower lobe received only 13% of total lung perfusion and only 5.5% of total lung ventilation.

In an Italian multicenter study, the authors evaluated the effect of lobectomy performed for lung cancer on pulmonary function in patients who had chronic obstructive pulmonary disease.[9] Forty-nine patients who had normal pulmonary function tests were compared with 88 patients who had COPD. In patients who had a COPD index greater than 1.5, the postoperative FEV_1 and FEV_1/FVC decreased significantly, whereas in patients who had a COPD index less than 1.5, the postoperative FEV_1/FVC increased significantly and the FEV_1 remained unchanged. In patients who had RV and functional residual capacity greater than 115%, the postoperative FEV_1 diminished less compared with patients who had RV and functional residual capacity less than 115%. The study found that the observed postoperative FEV_1 was better than the predicted postoperative FEV_1 (ie, higher observed postoperative FEV_1/predicted postoperative FEV_1 ratio) in patients who had preoperative FEV_1/FVC of less than 55%, in whom the preoperative FEV_1 was less than 80% of predicted and the COPD index was less than 1.5. The authors concluded that patients who have mild to severe COPD could have a better late preservation of pulmonary function after lobectomy than healthy patients if appropriately evaluated and selected.

It can be seen that various groups have reported on different methods of patient evaluation and selection for offering patients to undergo a concomitant lung cancer resection and LVRS. Some of these studies have correlated preoperative ventilation function to postoperative ventilation and outcomes. Despite these various reported methods, no single test has been found to best define the patients who will and will not tolerate resection. Instead, the various investigations and evaluative processes, together with the physical condition of the patient and the surgeon's experience, help to select patients suitable for combined surgical resection to achieve optimal outcomes.

SUMMARY

Patients who are offered concomitant surgery are highly selected and must satisfy the strict criteria set out for both LVRS and cancer surgery. Several evaluative processes have been reported for the selection of suitable patients. These various evaluative processes, together with the physical condition of the patient and the surgeon's experience, help to best select patients suitable for combined surgical resection. Several intraoperative strategies are available for dealing with a patient who has concomitant lung cancer and severe emphysema. The choice of technique depends on the location and size of the tumor, the severity and distribution of the emphysema, and the surgeon's experience and preference. Lung volume reduction surgery in well-selected patients who have severe emphysema results in postoperative improvement of symptoms and measured pulmonary function. The combination of lung cancer resection with LVRS offers selected patients who have concomitant early lung cancer and severe emphysema the opportunity to undergo resection of their cancer with improvement rather than further reduction in their pulmonary function.[1] By traditional criteria these patients would otherwise be considered unsuitable surgical candidates because of the limited pulmonary function.

REFERENCES

1. Choong CK, Meyers BF, Battafarano RJ, et al. Lung cancer resection combined with lung volume reduction in patients with severe emphysema. J Thorac Cardiovasc Surg 2004;127:1323–31.
2. DeMeester SR, Patterson GA, Sundaresan RS, et al. Lobectomy combined with volume reduction for patients with lung cancer and advanced emphysema. J Thorac Cardiovasc Surg 1998;115:681–8.
3. McKenna RJ Jr, Fischel RJ, Brenner M, et al. Combined operations for lung volume reduction surgery and lung cancer. Chest 1996;110:885–8.
4. Korst RJ, Ginsberg RJ, Ailawadi M, et al. Lobectomy improves ventilatory function in selected patients with severe COPD. Ann Thorac Surg 1998;66:898–902.
5. Carretta A, Zannini P, Puglisi A, et al. Improvement of pulmonary function after lobectomy for non-small cell lung cancer in emphysematous patients. Eur J Cardiothorac Surg 1999;15:602–7.
6. Edwards JG, Duthie DJ, Waller DA. Lobar volume reduction surgery: a method of increasing the lung cancer resection rate in patients with emphysema. Thorax 2001;56:791–5.
7. Vaughan P, Oey I, Nakas A, et al. Is there a role for therapeutic lobectomy for emphysema? Eur J Cardiothorac Surg 2007;31:486–90.
8. Martin-Ucar AE, Fareed KR, Nakas A, et al. Is the initial feasibility of lobectomy for stage I non-small cell lung cancer in severe heterogeneous emphysema justified by long-term survival? Thorax 2007;62:577–80.
9. Baldi S, Ruffini E, Harari S, et al. Does lobectomy for lung cancer in patients with chronic obstructive pulmonary disease affect lung function? A multicenter national study. J Thorac Cardiovasc Surg 2005;130:1616–22.
10. Mentzer SJ, Swanson SJ. Treatment of patients with lung cancer and severe emphysema. Chest 1999;116:477S–9S.
11. Hayashi K, Fukushima K, Sagara Y, et al. Surgical treatment for patients with lung cancer complicated by severe pulmonary emphysema. Jpn J Thorac Cardiovasc Surg 1999;47:583–7.
12. Cesario A, Di Toro S, Granone P. Pulmonary lobectomy for cancer in patients with chronic obstructive pulmonary disease. J Thorac Cardiovasc Surg 2006;132:215–6.
13. Kushibe K, Takahama M, Tojo T, et al. Assessment of pulmonary function after lobectomy for lung cancer—upper lobectomy might have the same effect as lung volume reduction surgery. Eur J Cardiothorac Surg 2006;29:886–90.
14. Sekine Y, Iwata T, Chiyo M, et al. Minimal alteration of pulmonary function after lobectomy in lung cancer patients with chronic obstructive pulmonary disease. Ann Thorac Surg 2003;76:356–61.
15. Sinjan EA, Van Schil PE, Ortmanns P, et al. Improved ventilatory function after combined operation for pulmonary emphysema and lung cancer. Int Surg 1999;84:185–9.
16. DeRose JJ Jr, Argenziano M, El-Amir N, et al. Lung reduction operation and resection of pulmonary nodules in patients with severe emphysema. Ann Thorac Surg 1998;65:314–8.
17. Ohtsuka T, Kohno T, Nakajima J, et al. Thoracoscopic surgery for lung cancer complicated by emphysema in elderly patients. Report of three cases. Int Surg 1996;81:245–7.
18. Garzon JC, Ng CSH, Sihoe ADL, et al. Video-assisted thoracic surgery pulmonary resection for lung cancer in patients with poor lung function. Ann Thorac Surg 2006;81:1996–2003.
19. Subotic DR, Mandaric DV, Eminovic TM, et al. Influence of chronic obstructive pulmonary disease on postoperative lung function and complications in patients undergoing operations for primary non-small cell lung cancer. J Thorac Cardiovasc Surg 2007;134:1292–9.
20. Pompeo E, De Dominicis E, Ambrogi V, et al. Quality of life after tailored combined surgery for stage I non-small-cell lung cancer and severe emphysema. Ann Thorac Surg 2003;76:1821–7.
21. Ciccone AM, Meyers BF, Guthrie TJ, et al. Long-term outcome of bilateral lung volume reduction in 250 consecutive patients with emphysema. J Thorac Cardiovasc Surg 2003;125:513–25.
22. Cooper JD, Patterson GA, Sundaresan RS, et al. Results of 150 consecutive bilateral lung volume reduction procedures in patients with severe emphysema. J Thorac Cardiovasc Surg 1996;112:1319–29.
23. Meyers BF, Sultan PK, Guthrie TJ, et al. Outcomes after unilateral lung volume reduction. Ann Thorac Surg 2008;86:204–11.
24. DeCamp MM Jr, Lipson D, Krasna M, et al. The evaluation and preparation of the patient for lung volume reduction surgery. Proc Am Thorac Soc 2008;4:427–31.
25. DeCamp MM Jr, McKenna RJ Jr, Deschamps CC, et al. Lung volume reduction surgery: technique,

operative mortality, and morbidity. Proc Am Thorac Soc 2008;5:442–6.

26. Washko GR, Hoffman E, Reilly JJ. Radiographic evaluation of the potential lung volume reduction surgery candidate. Proc Am Thorac Soc 2008;5: 421–6.

27. The National Emphysema Treatment Trial Research Group. Rationale and design of the National Emphysema Treatment Trial (NETT): a prospective randomized trial of lung volume reduction surgery. J Thorac Cardiovasc Surg 1999;118:518–28.

28. Naunheim KS, Wood DE, Krasna MJ, et al. Predictors of operative mortality and cardiopulmonary morbidity in the National Emphysema Treatment Trial. J Thorac Cardiovasc Surg 2006;131:43–53.

29. Scott WJ, Howington J, Feigenberg S, et al. American College of Chest Physicians. Treatment of non-small cell lung cancer stage I and stage II:

ACCP evidence-based clinical practice guidelines. Chest 2007;132:234S–42S.

30. Robinson LA, Ruckdeschel JC, Wagner H Jr, et al. American College of Chest Physicians. Treatment of non-small cell lung cancer-stage IIIA: ACCP evidence-based clinical practice guidelines. Chest 2007;132:243S–65S.

31. Naunheim KS, Wood DE, Mohsenifar Z, et al. The National Emphysema Treatment Trial Research Group. Long-term follow-up of patients receiving lung-volume-reduction surgery versus medical therapy for severe emphysema by the National Emphysema Treatment Trial Research Group. Ann Thorac Surg 2006;82:431–43.

32. Fishman A, Martinez F, Naunheim K, et al. A randomized trial comparing LVRS with medical therapy for severe emphysema. N Engl J Med 2003;348: 2059–73.

Combined Cardiac and Lung Volume Reduction Surgery

Cliff K. Choong, MBBS, FRACS, FRCS[a,b,]*, Ralph A. Schmid, MD[c],
Daniel L. Miller, MD[d], Julian A. Smith, MB, MS, FRACS, FACS, FCSANZ[b]

KEYWORDS

- Cardiac • Coronary • Valve • Surgery • Emphysema
- Lung volume reduction

Coronary artery disease (CAD) is prevalent in patients who have severe emphysema and who are being considered for lung volume reduction surgery (LVRS).[1] Significant valvular heart diseases may also coexist in these patients. The National Emphysema Treatment Trial excludes patients who have a variety of cardiovascular risk factors from undergoing LVRS,[2] as do many surgeons who perform the procedure outside of the trial. Few thoracic surgeons have performed LVRS in patients who have severe cardiac diseases. Conversely, few cardiac surgeons have been willing to undertake major cardiac surgery in patients who have severe emphysema. This report reviews the evidence regarding combined cardiac surgery and LVRS to determine the optimal management strategy for patients who have severe emphysema and who are suitable for LVRS, but who also have coexisting significant cardiac diseases that are operable.

LITERATURE REVIEW

There are few reports on combined cardiac surgery and LVRS (**Table 1**).[3–9] Patients are highly selected who have criteria suitable for them to undergo LVRS and also have cardiac diseases that in general require straightforward cardiac surgery. The combined procedures have been performed using a median sternotomy that allows for a standard cardiac surgical approach and also provides access to both pleural spaces for bilateral LVRS. The operative strategy adopted in majority of the cases has been to perform the cardiac procedure first, followed by bilateral LVRS (see **Table 1**). The LVRS is performed after termination of cardiopulmonary bypass support (CPB), full reversal of heparin, and determination of satisfactory cardiorespiratory stability. Of the 20 patients under consideration in **Table 1**, all apart from one patient survived the combined procedure and experienced marked symptomatic improvements on follow-up.[3–9]

DISCUSSION

Most patients who have end-stage emphysema have a history of smoking and are therefore at increased risk for CAD. Turnheer and colleagues[1] reported that 15% percent of the 124 patients who were considered suitable to undergo LVRS in their study were found to have coexisting CAD. Because dyspnea is often multifactorial, some patients have severe and disabling symptoms as the result of a combination of cardiac and pulmonary diseases. If untreated,

[a] Papworth Hospital NHS Foundation Trust and Department of Surgery, The University of Cambridge, Cambridge, UK
[b] Department of Surgery, Monash University, Level 5, Block E, Monash Medical Centre, 246 Clayton Road, Melbourne, Victoria 3168, Australia
[c] Division of General Thoracic Surgery, University Hospital Berne, Berne, Switzerland
[d] General Thoracic Surgery, Division of Cardiothoracic Surgery, Department of Surgery, Emory University School of Medicine, Emory University Hospital, Atlanta, GA, USA
* Corresponding author. Department of Surgery, Monash University, Level 5, Block E, Monash Medical Centre, 246 Clayton Road, Melbourne, Victoria 3168, Australia.
E-mail address: cliffchoong@hotmail.com (C.K. Choong).

Thorac Surg Clin 19 (2009) 217–221
doi:10.1016/j.thorsurg.2009.04.001
1547-4127/09/$ – see front matter © 2009 Elsevier Inc. All rights reserved.

Table 1
Literature review of combined cardiac and lung volume reduction surgery

Authors	No. of Patients	Types of Cardiac Procedure[a]	Timing of Bilateral LVRS	Operative Time	Timing of Postoperative Extubation	Complications	Postoperative Day of Chest Tube Removal	Day of Discharge Following Surgery	Follow-up
Miller et al.[3]	10	All patients had CABG; median no. of grafts was three	Following termination of CPB and reversal of heparin	Median CPB time was 58 minutes	Nine patients extubated within 12 hours	No major complications	Not reported	Median hospital stay 10 days (range 7–21 days)	Well at 6 months with marked improvements
Whyte et al.[4]	1	CABG × 3 and MV repair	Before CPB	Not reported	Day 1	Not reported	Day 4	Day 8	Well at 3 months with marked improvements
Oto et al.[5]	1	CABG × 3	During CPB	Not reported	12 hours	Ischemic bowel and sepsis leading to death on day 5	Not applicable	Not applicable	Not applicable
Schmid et al.[6]	2	CABG × 5	Unilateral LVRS performed for diffuse emphysema during CPB	Not reported	Not specified for this patient	Not specified for this patient	Not specified for this patient	Discharged date not specified for this patient	Not reported
		AVR	Following AVR	Not reported	Extubated on day 12	Pulmonary hypertension and unilateral pneumonia	Not reported	Day 28	Well at 3 months

Study	n	Cardiac procedure		Mean operative time	Extubation	Complications		Mean length of stay	Outcome
Shrager et al.[7]	4	CABG ×1 CABG ×2 CABG ×2 AVR	For three patients, following termination of CPB and reversal of heparin; for one patient, while still on CPB	Mean operative time was 207 minutes	1 patient extubated in the operating room; remaining patients at a mean of 14 hours	No major complications; five minor complications	Three patients were discharged with Heimlich valves; mean time of chest tube removal was 11.5 days	Mean length of stay was 9.8 days	All patients well at a mean follow-up of 22.8 months with symptomatic improvements
Choong et al.[8]	1	AVR	Following termination of CPB and reversal of heparin	Not reported	Early extubation in ICU	No major complication	Day 4	Day 8	Well at 4 months with marked improvements
Choong et al.[9]	1	CABG ×1	Following termination of CPB and reversal of heparin	Not reported	Early extubation in ICU	No major complication	Day 5	Day 9	Well at 6 months with marked improvements

Abbreviations: AVR, aortic valve replacement; CABG, coronary artery bypass graft; CPB, cardiopulmonary bypass support; ICU, intensive care unit; MV, mitral valve.
[a] All the cardiac procedures were performed using cardiopulmonary bypass support.

symptomatic cardiac diseases are associated with a poor prognosis.[10,11] The National Emphysema Treatment Trial (NETT) has shown that in highly selected patients, LVRS can offer greater symptomatic and prognostic benefits than for patients who are treated using maximal medical therapy alone.[12,13] Although many candidates for LVRS have CAD that may be amenable to the use of percutaneous intervention, others have cardiac diseases that are not appropriate for such intervention and require cardiac surgery. Options for the latter patients include foregoing LVRS, performing LVRS and the cardiac procedure as a staged operation at separate anesthetic settings, or combining the two procedures in a single operation.

Although the literature on combining cardiac procedures and pulmonary resections for patients who have cancer is extensive, there is little information regarding the use of combined cardiac surgery and LVRS. It may be that few thoracic surgeons are willing to offer LVRS for patients who have coexisting significant cardiac disease because that has traditionally been considered one of the standard criteria for exclusion. Of the 511 patients in the non–high-risk group of the National Emphysema Treatment Trial who underwent LVRS, pulmonary morbidity occurred in 29.8% and cardiovascular morbidity occurred in 20.0% of the patients, with an operative mortality rate of 5.5%.[14]

The presence of significant cardiac disease increases the risk for morbidity and mortality associated with pulmonary surgery. These increased risks are likely to be even more important after an operation such as LVRS, which severely stresses patients who begin with compensated cardiopulmonary function. Referring physicians are also less likely to refer emphysematous patients who have significant cardiac diseases for surgical evaluation because of the presence of both diseases. There may also be an underreporting of such combined cases because of either unsuccessful outcomes or a lack of manuscript submission, even in successful cases.

A number of authors have now shown that in highly selected patients, a combined cardiac surgery and LVRS procedure is feasible, can be done safely, and can result in improvements in pulmonary function similar to those reported after isolated LVRS procedures.[3–9] The fact that cardiac operations can be performed safely in conjunction with lung volume reduction has implications for two groups of patients who have severe emphysema:[1] those who are denied LVRS on the basis of concomitant cardiac disease and[2] those who are denied a cardiac operation because of a perceived excessive operative risk secondary to concomitant severe emphysema. The first group of patients includes those who have historically been turned down for LVRS because of concomitant valvular or coronary disease that would either increase the patients' risks from LVRS or limit their potential for full postoperative rehabilitation and recovery. In the second group of patients, evaluation of suitability for LVRS may indicate that a combined operation may not only be feasible but may actually reduce the risks from the cardiac procedure by decreasing postoperative pulmonary complications. Combined operations have produced excellent functional results, with both disease processes being significantly treated.[3,4,6–9]

There are a number of advantages in performing a combined operation. First, patient convenience is improved. A combined operation requires a single hospital admission, the use of a single general anesthetic, and a single hospital stay. Second, difficulties that are associated with performing the operations as a staged procedure are avoided. An example is avoiding the risks in redoing a sternotomy to perform the LVRS as a second procedure. Even if a surgeon is performing a video-assisted thoracoscopic LVRS after a CABG procedure, there are likely to be adhesions related to the previous opening of the pleura to harvest the internal mammary artery for use as a conduit. Pleural adhesions can make LVRS difficult and are associated with increased morbidity. Third, combining the operations, with a single hospital admission, reduces costs.

Multidisciplinary strategies are important in achieving a successful outcome in the management of these high-risk patients.[8,9] A skilled anesthetist is required to ensure the proper placement of an epidural catheter and double-lumen endotracheal tube and careful intraoperative management of the patient. An error in any of these areas could lead to severe consequences. Because of the impending full anticoagulation required for CPB, some anesthetists are unwilling to place an epidural catheter for fear of a resulting epidural hemorrhage. In cases in which the operative team elects to place an epidural catheter, the placement should be carried out at least 4 hours before the scheduled surgery, a strategy that has been shown to be safe despite full anticoagulation for CPB.[15] The use of postoperative thoracic epidural analgesia can contribute to a patient's good compliance with physiotherapy and breathing exercises, thereby reducing the risks of postoperative sputum retention and chest infection. Careful postoperative intensive care management by an experienced intensivist is important in the maintenance of cardiorespiratory stability. A planned early extubation helps to minimize the risks associated with mechanical ventilation. Daily medical management by a chest physician in the perioperative period will also ensure that the patient receives optimal medical therapy for the emphysematous disease.[8,9] The surgical strategy of performing the cardiac procedure first followed by reversal of anticoagulation before LVRS will ensure that there is normal hemostasis during LVRS to minimize the risk for pulmonary hemorrhage.[3,5–9] There is a potential increased risk for pulmonary hemorrhage in performing LVRS before or during CPB because of the full anticoagulation required for CPB. The strategy of performing LVRS following the cardiac procedure also allows for pleural adhesions to be divided while both lungs are deflated during CPB. Apart from minimizing the risk for pulmonary contusion, this strategy also allows the surgeon to see the lungs in the incompletely deflated state, which highlights gas-retaining target areas. It is important that satisfactory cardiorespiratory stability and hemostasis are achieved before performing the LVRS. These multidisciplinary strategies have allowed for successful combined operations and outcomes.[8,9] It is critical, however, that patients being considered for combined cardiac surgery and LVRS be excellent candidates for both operations because a less-than-optimal outcome from one procedure may mitigate any benefits brought about by the other procedure. This surgical strategy should preferably be undertaken in centers that have staff members with a large body of experience in the surgical management of patients who have both cardiac and pulmonary diseases, such as centers with staff members accustomed to performing LVRS.

In summary, a combined cardiac operation and LVRS can be done safely in highly selected patients, with improvements in pulmonary function similar to those reported after isolated LVRS procedures. A multidisciplinary team approach is important in achieving a successful outcome in these patients.

REFERENCES

1. Turnheer R, Muntwhyler J, Stammberger U, et al. Coronary artery disease in patients undergoing lung volume reduction surgery for emphysema. Chest 1997;112:122–8.
2. The National Emphysema Treatment Trial Research Group. Rationale and design of the National Emphysema Treatment Trial (NETT): a prospective randomized trial of lung volume reduction surgery. J Thorac Cardiovasc Surg 1999;118:518–28.
3. Miller DL, Dowling RD, Slater AD, et al. Combined lung volume reduction and coronary artery bypass surgery. Chest 1996;110(Suppl 49S):49–50.
4. Whyte RI, Bria W, Martinez FJ, et al. Combined lung volume reduction and mitral valve reconstruction. Ann Thorac Surg 1998;66:1414–6.
5. Oto O, Hazan E, Silistreli E, et al. Lung volume reduction in parallel with coronary heart surgery: a case report. J Int Med Res 1998;26:266–9.
6. Schmid RA, Stammberger U, Hillinger S, et al. Lung volume reduction surgery combined with cardiac interventions. Eur J Cardiothorac Surg 1999;15:585–91.
7. Shrager JB, Kozyak BW, Roberts JR, et al. Successful experience with simultaneous lung volume reduction and cardiac procedures. J Thorac Cardiovasc Surg 2001;122:196–7.
8. Choong CK, Agarwal A, Pulimood T, et al. Concomitant bilateral lung volume reduction surgery and aortic valve replacement: multidisciplinary strategies in achieving a successful outcome. J Thorac Cardiovasc Surg, in press.
9. Choong CK, J Naylor, Vuylsteke A, et al. Successful combined bilateral lung volume reduction and coronary artery bypass grafting surgery: implications and advantages. J Thorac Cardiovasc Surg, in press.
10. Schawrz F, Baumann P, Manthey J, et al. The effect of aortic valve replacement on survival. Circulation 1982;66:1105–10.
11. Morrow DA, Gersh BJ, Braunwald E, et al. Chronic coronary artery disease. In: Zipes DP, Libby P, Bonow RO, editors. Braunwald's heart disease. 7th edition. Philadelphia: Elsevier Saunders; 2005. p. 1281–354.
12. Fishman A, Martinez F, Naunheim K, et al. National Emphysema Treatment Trial Research Group. A randomized trial comparing lung-volume-reduction surgery with medical therapy for severe emphysema. N Engl J Med 2003;348(21):2059–73.
13. Naunheim KS, Wood DE, Mohsenifar Z, et al. National Emphysema Treatment Trial Research Group. Long-term follow-up of patients receiving lung-volume-reduction surgery versus medical therapy for severe emphysema by the National Emphysema Treatment Trial Research Group. Ann Thorac Surg 2006;82:431–43.
14. Naunheim KS, Wood DE, Krasna MJ, et al. National Emphysema Treatment Trial Research Group. Predictors of operative mortality and cardiopulmonary morbidity in the National Emphysema Treatment Trial. J Thorac Cardiovasc Surg 2006;131:43–53.
15. Chaney MA. Intrathecal and epidural anesthesia and analgesia for cardiac surgery. Anesth Analg 2006;102:45–64.

Intraoperative and Postoperative Management of Air Leaks in Patients with Emphysema

Joseph B. Shrager, MD[a,b,*], Malcolm M. DeCamp, MD[c], Sudish C. Murthy, MD, PhD[d]

KEYWORDS

- Lung • Pulmonary • Lung resection
- Chronic obstructive pulmonary disease
- Lung volume reduction surgery • Bronchopleural fistula

Parenchymal air leaks (AL) that occur after pulmonary resection are among the most common perioperative problems that thoracic surgeons are called upon to manage. Although most ALs seal spontaneously within a few days and cause no clinical sequelae, it appears clear in the literature that ALs as a whole significantly increase morbidity and costs.[1–5] When ALs are large or persist (becoming a prolonged air leak or PAL), they grow in importance from simply serving as a nuisance to the patient and surgeon to potentially leading to serious problems including respiratory compromise, atelectasis, pneumonia, and empyema. Rarely, PAL may require reoperation. These prolonged and complicated ALs occur most commonly in patients who have substantial emphysema.

Although there has been increasing attention devoted to the study of ALs and their management by industry and academia in the past several years, the literature in the area remains in evolution. Much has been learned about the risk factors, natural history, and evolving treatment of ALs, but much remains to be learned. For example, multiple methods to manage ALs have been proposed, and some of these have been subjected to rigorous study, but the data on their utility are often conflicting. Further, it is clear that emphysema is a prime risk factor, but exactly what degree of emphysema places a patient at sufficiently high risk for a PAL to merit the use of expensive prophylactic materials or time-consuming intraoperative maneuvers remains uncertain.

This article begins with a brief review of the incidence and risk factors for ALs. It then breaks down the discussion of the prophylaxis and therapy of ALs into a section on intraoperative management of AL and one on pleural drain management, which discusses the most important issue in the postoperative management of routine, small ALs. This is followed by a section focused upon ALs in patients undergoing lung volume reduction surgery (LVRS), perhaps those most at risk for complicated or prolonged ALs. The article closes with a discussion of the management options for PALs.

[a] Division of Thoracic Surgery, Department of Cardiothoracic Surgery, Stanford University School of Medicine, Stanford Hospitals and Clinics, 2nd Floor, Falk Building, 300 Pasteur Drive, Stanford, CA 94305-5407, USA
[b] Veterans Affairs Palo Alto Health Care System, Palo Alto, CA, USA
[c] Division of Cardiothoracic Surgery, Department of Surgery, Harvard Medical School, Beth Israel Deaconess Medical Center, 185 Pilgrim Road, Deaconess 201, Boston, MA 02215, USA
[d] Department of Thoracic and Cardiovascular Surgery, Center of Major Airway Disease, Cleveland Clinic, 9500 Euclid Avenue, Desk F24, Cleveland, OH 44195, USA
* Corresponding author. Division of Thoracic Surgery, Department of Cardiothoracic Surgery, Stanford University School of Medicine, Stanford Hospitals and Clinics, 2nd Floor, Falk Building, 300 Pasteur Drive, Stanford, CA 94305-5407.
E-mail address: shrager@stanford.edu (J.B. Shrager).

Thorac Surg Clin 19 (2009) 223–231
doi:10.1016/j.thorsurg.2009.02.004
1547-4127/09/$ – see front matter. Published by Elsevier Inc.

INCIDENCE OF AIR LEAKS

An AL of any size or duration has been reported to be present in between 28% and 60% of the broad population of patients undergoing routine pulmonary resection.[1,2] A PAL, variably defined as a leak persisting beyond postoperative day (POD) 5 or POD 7, occurs in 8% to 26% of these patients.[1,5–8] Within the National Emphysema Treatment Trial (NETT), an AL occurred at some point in 90% of bilateral LVRS patients; the median duration of AL was 7 days, and 12% had a persistent AL even at 30 days postoperatively.[4] Twenty-two percent of similar patients with severe emphysema undergoing non-LVRS pulmonary resection had an AL lasting beyond 7 days in one group's experience.[9]

RISK FACTORS FOR AIR LEAKS

Many studies have evaluated factors associated with PAL following pulmonary resection, and the one risk factor that is identified most repeatedly and convincingly is the degree of chronic obstructive pulmonary disease (COPD). Although studies do not generally separate out COPD patients who have predominately chronic bronchitis from those who have predominately parenchymal destruction caused by emphysema, it is highly likely that it is those on the emphysema end of the COPD spectrum that are at highest risk. It appears that the fragile lung tissue of emphysema patients is prone to develop tears and thus ALs from staple lines and areas adjacent to staple lines, from areas of dissection within the fissures, and from areas where retraction upon adhesions may cause parenchymal injury. Preoperative tests that reflect severity of COPD and are associated with PAL include postoperative predicted forced expiratory volume in 1 second (FEV$_1$), FEV$_1$ less than 79% predicted,[9] FEV$_1$ less than 1.5 L, and FEV$_1$ and FEV$_1$/forced vital capacity (FVC) ratio both less than 70%.[8,10–12]

Other risk factors that are not direct reflections of degree of emphysema but which have been associated with PAL include:

Diffusing capacity of the lung for carbon monoxide (DLCO) less than 80% predicted[8]
The presence of adhesions[10]
Upper lobectomy and bilobectomy versus other types of lobectomy[10]
Lobectomy versus lesser resections[5]
Presence of a pneumothorax coinciding with the AL[5,8]
Chronic oral steroid use[5]
Leak of size 4 or greater on the scale of 1 to 7 proposed by Cerfolio and colleagues[5]

Factors about which one might be concerned about but are not associated with PAL in most studies include: preoperative chemotherapy,[7,12] age,[5,7,13] status of interlobar fissures,[5,7] and nutritional status.[8,12] The specific risk factors in LVRS patients will be discussed.

INTRAOPERATIVE MANAGEMENT OF AIR LEAK

It is becoming apparent that AL following lung resection should be considered in the same context as intraoperative blood loss; that is, there is no amount of AL that is ever good. To this end, there have been several strategies developed to combat this problem. Before delving into specifics, it is perhaps best to remember that a premium must be placed on careful handling of the lung, meticulous dissection of the fissure (for lobectomy), and avoidance of denuding visceral pleural surfaces by carefully lysing pleural adhesions.

Because every attempt should be made to leave the operating room with pneumostasis, vigorous interrogation of such should be performed at the conclusion of the operation. Controlled reinflation of the lung is important during this process, as hyperinflation and barotrauma may occur and promote AL. Certainly no more than 25 cm of pressure should be exerted in lung reinflation, and the authors have found that 20 cm is adequate and perhaps safer. Unfortunately, even when a thorough evaluation is performed and no evidence of AL is found intraoperatively, there is a surprisingly high incidence of AL noted in the early perioperative period.[14]

Intraoperative management of AL should be directed toward three primary endpoints: prevention, repair, and providing favorable conditions for early perioperative resolution. Once again, there is nothing that can replace good surgical judgment in these circumstances, as a very large AL after a complex wedge resection, or even LVRS, sometimes will be handled best with completion lobectomy instead of attempted repair.

Air Leak Prevention

Buttressing of parenchymal staple lines has been documented. Various materials have been studied, and there are no data to suggest an obvious advantage of a biologic material compared with a synthetic such as polytetrafluoroethylene (PTFE). Buttresses reinforce the margin longitudinally and compress the base of the staple line, presumably reducing the chance of staple line dehiscence during re-expansion or vigorous cough, and reducing the possibility of leaking directly through staple holes. It is also theoretically possible, however, that they could promote AL by causing high surface tension in the region immediately subjacent to the margin because of excessive compression of the staple line itself. Thus the need for clinical studies to establish efficacy.

Choice of patients upon whom to use this costly strategy is critical. Most would concur that buttresses should be considered for patients who have moderately severe or severe emphysema, with specific emphasis given to patients who have LVRS or others who have emphysema undergoing nonanatomic wedge resections. Surprisingly, buttressing of any type did not appear to impact AL within the NETT study's nonrandomized analysis of this subject.[4] Nonetheless, there are randomized data that demonstrate an advantage from buttressing staple lines during LVRS.[15,16] Despite these data favoring use in patients who have LVRS, it is not clear whether the additional costs are justifiable in patients who have less diseased lung or those undergoing lobectomy. Several small studies offer conflicting data on this topic. In this circumstance, emphysema patients who have incomplete or difficult fissures undergoing lobectomy, or patients who have emphysema undergoing segmental resections, might be appropriate candidates for buttressing.

Topical sealants can be considered as a preventative or a reparative measure. Numerous biologic and synthetic agents have been developed, and many have been included in randomized trials.[17–20] It is difficult to assess efficacy of one sealant versus another, and only a handful of individual trials have showed statistically significant reductions in AL. When reviewed cumulatively, however, there appears to be a general reduction of AL with the use of sealants. Sealants can be applied to staple lines regardless of leak testing (preventative) or only after a leak is identified (reparative). Most have been tested on patients undergoing anatomic resection without identification of patients at particular risk for AL, and seldom after wedge resection. Consequently, it is difficult to speculate on the impact of sealants in what might be considered a high-risk population, and understanding this is warranted given what would be the additional costs incurred by their routine use.

Air Leak Repair

Although small leaks almost always will seal spontaneously within 2 or 3 days of operation, when larger ALs are identified intraoperatively, repair should be considered. In addition to use of a topical sealant, this might consist of something as simple and inexpensive as a horizontal mattress suture to coapt a visceral pleural defect or a buttressed restapling. Autologous tissues, including the pleura, pericardium, or pericardial fat pad, can be used as biologic pledgets.[21] Teflon or felt pledgets also may be useful in these situations. These pledgets are particularly useful when the quality of the lung tissue is poor (emphysema) and unlikely to support simple suturing.

Healing of ALs is thought to be facilitated by pleural–pleural apposition, and this is supported by the finding that pneumothorax is a risk factor for PAL.[5] Several intraoperative strategies designed to reduce the space within the operated hemithorax have been developed and serve as important adjuncts to AL management. Because not all ALs are detectable intraoperatively, the use of these techniques may be extended to include application after any resection resulting in a large unfilled space within the chest, regardless of the presence of AL.

Initially, the lung should be released completely from all parietal pleural attachments. The inferior pulmonary ligament should be divided up to the inferior pulmonary vein and anterior and posterior pleural reflections of the hilum dissected. Any adhesions should be lysed and the lung fully mobilized from diaphragmatic surface to cupula.

A simple technique to transiently reduce the functional size of the pleural cavity is to anesthetize the phrenic nerve. This is recommended only for patients who have near-normal preoperative pulmonary function. The phrenic neurovascular pedicle is grasped gently as it courses above the hilum with a Babcock clamp and 1 to 2 cc of 0.5% bupivicaine (without epinephrine) are injected as a wheal around the pedicle but not through the pericardium. The nerve is not injected directly, and crushing the pedicle in not advocated. The immediate postoperative chest radiogram will demonstrate an elevated ipsilateral hemidiaphragm that resumes a more normal contour over the ensuing 24 hours. The elevated hemidiaphragm will promote early pleural–pleural apposition and will reduce the amount of free space within the hemithorax.

Another simple strategy is to leave basilar and apical chest tubes within the hemithorax. This serves to control the space completely. Applying low suction (10 to 20 cm H_2O) for 24 to 48 hours may help coapt the pleural surfaces, although the benefit of suction over water seal in the absence of a large AL is unclear, as discussed in other sections of this article.

Dissection of the parietal pleura off of the endothoracic fascia is another useful adjunct to help fill an anticipated space following lung resection. This is performed primarily as a pleural tent, where the pleura is dissected intact off the endothoracic fascia, usually beginning at the site of a thoracotomy or thoracostomy incision and proceeding in a cephalad direction. The pleura must be mobilized completely from the apex of the chest cavity. The pleural flap then is draped over the top of the lung. Chest drains are placed within the tent but not to the apex of the hemithorax to prevent elevating the tent away from the top of the lung. Pleural fluid generally accumulates between the endothoracic fascia and the tent, thereby effectively reducing the volume of the chest.

It has been suggested that a pleural tent should accompany every upper lobectomy.[22,23] Although this is supported by some randomized data, the creation of an effective tent is not a trivial undertaking, and in some patients it is not even possible. Dense pleural adhesions may compromise the ability to create an intact tent. Moreover, some parietal pleural envelopes are simply too thin to permit easy mobilization. As would be expected, hemothorax is a possible complication. Like most other intraoperative adjuncts, pleural tenting likely is best reserved for patients undergoing upper lobectomy who are at greatest risk for a troublesome AL, those who have substantial emphysema.

There is little information to support routine use of pleural tenting after LVRS. Although this would seem to be a useful adjunct in this setting, it is somewhat cumbersome to develop a pleural tent through a sternotomy exposure. From a lateral approach (video-assisted thoracic surgical, VATS), however, the tent is much easier to create. If possible, tenting would be favored during LVRS, although there are no published data with comparison groups to support this.

For the uncommon situation where a basilar space needs to be controlled, what might be called a pleural rug can be constructed similarly. This is useful for AL after decortication in conditions where the lung does not have enough compliance to fill the lower chest cavity. The parietal pleura is thickened universally in these types of cases and can be mobilized off the lateral chest wall and sewn directly to the dome of the diaphragm to obliterate the costophrenic sulcus.

Pneumatic resuspension of the diaphragm (pneumoperitoneum) is another useful technique to reduce the size of the chest cavity. It has been trialed after lower lobectomy and bilobectomy and entails instilling 1000 to 1500 cc of air directly across the diaphragm intraoperatively.[24,25] Although data are limited, there seems to be reduced prevalence of AL and shorter length of stay in treated patients. From a technical standpoint, the procedure is performed using an extended 16- or 18-gauge catheter

placed directly across the diaphragm (and secured with a purse string suture), and the air is instilled gradually up to the target volume. There will be a noticeable rise in the dome of the diaphragm. After the catheter is removed and the chest closed, the patient should be maintained in a head-of-bed elevated, semidecubitus position with the operated side up in an attempt to keep as much air under the ipsilateral diaphragm as possible for the first 24 to 48 hours. Most patients tolerate the procedure quite well, although complaints of abdominal bloating are not uncommon. When a large space (approximately 30%), exists after a lower or bilobectomy, or when a large AL persists after reparative measures, creation of pneumoperitoneum should be considered.

Thoracoplasty and muscle flap transposition are more extreme measures to reduce the size of the chest and are seldom applicable at an initial operation. They are more commonly used in the rare instance that reoperation is required for persistent AL.

Although not well-studied, occasionally, a mechanical pleurodesis or pleurectomy will be a useful adjunct for AL control or prevention when the development of a space is not an issue. The circumstance most commonly encountered where this might be useful is that of a wedge resection for nodulectomy or lung biopsy. In patients who have suspected impaired wound healing (eg, steroid dependency, neutropenia), a local mechanical abrasion may add a measure of security to allow for early and permanent annealing of the stapled margin to the chest wall. This technique also can be useful for patients who have respiratory failure and interstitial lung disease undergoing open lung (or VATS) biopsy. These patients are, perhaps, at the greatest risk for a protracted alveolar AL, because they present with noncompliant lung that is difficult to staple, and they often have a postoperative requirement for extended positive pressure ventilation.

POSTOPERATIVE MANAGEMENT OF AIR LEAK
Pleural Drain Management

Despite the absence of rigorous evidence to support the practice, since at least the 1960s most surgeons have placed chest drains to -20 cm H_2O suction following pulmonary resections, converting the tubes to water seal only when there is no visible AL. This practice appears to be based upon the belief that apposition between the visceral and parietal pleurae is the most important factor in helping to seal leaks and the greater likelihood of achieving this apposition with the application of some level of suction.

It is also possible, however, that achieving pleural–pleural apposition is less important in allowing leaks to seal than is minimizing the volume of air flowing through a visceral pleural defect. The latter might be achieved by minimizing the use of suction. It was suggested first in patients who had LVRS that placing patients' chest tubes to the traditional −20 cm suction might prolong ALs.[26,27] Most surgeons performing LVRS now manage chest drains in these patients with water seal alone, and this change in management appears to have played a role in significant reductions in morbidity and mortality following LVRS. This experience with LVRS stimulated surgeons to study whether various water seal algorithms would reduce AL/PAL following non-LVRS pulmonary resections and in patients who had lesser degrees of emphysema or no substantial emphysema.

Five prospective, randomized trials evaluating various early water seal algorithms have been published (**Table 1**) and several other retrospective or nonrandomized reports. Of the five prospective, randomized studies, three found a benefit to early water seal; one found no difference between water seal and suction approaches, and one found water seal to be slightly detrimental. In the first study,[28] patients who had an AL present on the morning of POD 2 were randomized to either remain on −20 suction (n=15) or be placed to water seal (n=18). In the water seal group, 67% of the ALs sealed by POD 3, while in the suction group only 7% sealed (P=.001). In the next study,[29] a water seal protocol that removed patients from suction immediately after leaving the operating room was compared with continued -20 suction. There was a significant reduction in AL duration (1.50 versus 3.27 days; P=.05; P=.02 if corrected for length of staple line) in the water seal group, but there was no significant reduction in length of stay (although shorter in the water seal group; P=.18). Brunelli and colleagues,[10] in a larger randomized study that was a pure group of 145 lobectomy patients, found no benefit to water seal and in fact a slightly (but not significantly) higher cardiopulmonary complication rate in those placed to water seal on POD 1. In response to this finding, Brunelli's group[30] subsequently evaluated a modified protocol termed "alternate suction" that involved applying −10 cm suction during the night and water seal during the day beginning on POD 1. They felt that this might combine the benefits of suction (pleural apposition) and water seal (reducing the volume of air leaking through the parenchyma, simplifying early ambulation). With this protocol, they found no difference in the duration of AL or rate of cardiopulmonary complications between the "alternate suction"

and water seal groups, but there was shorter chest tube duration (P=.002), shorter hospital stay (P=.004), and fewer PALs (P=.02) in the alternate suction group. Finally, Alphonso and colleagues[31] performed a still larger study (n=239) comparing patients randomized to suction versus water seal immediately in the operating room without even a brief period of suction. No difference was found in Kaplan-Meier analysis of AL duration, the only end point reported.

Among those studies that routinely obtained chest radiograms after placement to water seal and reported on pneumothorax rates, approximately 25% of patients developed a pneumothorax of sufficient size to require placement back to −10 or −20 cm suction. None of these pneumothoraces, however, were clinically important, and no patients developed clinically significant postoperative spaces or pleural effusions. It may, in fact, be the lack of routine chest radiograms in the first Brunelli study that led to the slightly increased complication rate. There are criticisms that can be leveled at any of these studies (eg, the Cerfolio and Marshall studies included some sublobar resections, so it is difficult to reach conclusions about lobectomy patients from them).

Still, the authors believe that the balance of the evidence indicates that there is value to reducing suction below the traditional −20 cm, even while an air leak persists, in most patients following lobectomy or sublobar resection. The ideal reduced suction algorithm, however, is uncertain. Available evidence supports using a brief period (either in the operating room only or overnight) of −10 cm suction followed by water seal in patients who have less than a large AL. As long as a sizeable pneumothorax, progressive subcutaneous emphysema, or clinical deterioration does not develop, water seal could be maintained until chest tube removal. Optimal management with this protocol mandates at least one chest radiogram several hours after being placed to water seal. Certainly, one would not want to use early water seal in patients with restrictive lung disease who likely would require some degree of suction to promote re-expansion in the face of an AL, and it also might be contraindicated to use early water seal if it is felt that there is an unusual risk of postoperative bleeding.

PROPHYLAXIS AND MANAGEMENT OF AIR LEAKS FOLLOWING LUNG VOLUME REDUCTION SURGERY

LVRS as a primary treatment for symptomatic emphysema was reintroduced into the general thoracic surgery lexicon by Cooper and

Table 1
Randomized prospective trials evaluating early water seal algorithms

Author	Algorithm Evaluated	N	Resections Included	CXRs Obtained to Rule Out PTX	Benefit to Water Seal	Significant Benefits
Cerfolio[28]	Water seal on POD 2 after −20 cm	33	Lobectomy and sublobar	Yes	Yes	Greater AL sealing by POD 3
Marshall[29]	Water seal after −20 cm only while in OR	68	Lobectomy and sublobar	Yes	Yes	Reduced AL duration
Brunelli[10]	Water seal on POD1 after −20 cm	145	Lobectomy	No	No	Do not recommend water seal since trend to increased complications
Brunelli[30]	Alternating -10 cm (night) and water seal (day) on POD1 versus full-time water seal after −10 cm	94	Lobectomy	No	Yes (to alternating suction/water seal)	Shorter tube duration, LOS, less PALs versus full-time water seal
Alphonso[31]	Immediate water seal	239	Lobectomy and sublobar	No	Yes	Recommend water seal since no differences found and water seal promotes mobilization

Abbreviations: AL, air leak; CXRs, chest radiograms; LOS, length of stay; OR, operating room; PALs, prolonged air leaks; POD, postoperative day; PTX, pneumothorax.

colleagues[32] in the mid-1990s. A bilateral stapled approach to reduce upper lobe-predominant disease was associated with functional and quality-of-life improvement in most highly selected patients. PAL was common following the procedure and was the major driver of the hospital length of stay, which approached 2 weeks after the trans-sternal approach.[26] The Washington University Group advocated buttressing of staple lines with bovine pericardial strips and suggested an aggressive application of water seal soon after surgery to reduce the magnitude and duration of AL.[33] These encouraging nonrandomized, single-institution results obtained by means of sternotomy were replicated by McKenna and colleagues[34] with respect to spirometric improvement, operative mortality and morbidity including PAL, and length of stay using a bilateral VATS approach. Their technique also involved routine staple line buttressing. Based on these two large single institutional trials (n ≥ 150 patients each), buttressing the parenchymal staple line during LVRS became a nearly routine practice.[35]

Various products have been developed to buttress lung parenchyma. These include bovine pericardium (Synovis, St. Paul, Minnesota), expanded polytetrafluoroethylene (ePTFE) (WL Gore, Flagstaff, Arizona), and their biodegradable counter parts Veritas and Seamguard respectively. A bovine collagen material manufactured by Johnson & Johnson (New Brunswick, New Jersey) also has been used.

Scant data comparing buttressing materials or documenting their efficacy over a nonbuttressed procedure exist. Hazelrigg and Naunheim performed a two-institution randomized trial comparing no buttress (n=65) with bovine pericardium buttressing (n=58) during LVRS. The buttress group had a 2.5-day shorter duration of chest tube drainage, which drove a 2.8-day shorter hospital length of stay. Surprisingly this shorter hospital stay did not translate into cost savings.[16] Fewer than 10% of the 580 patients undergoing LVRS in NETT were unbuttressed, making a buttressed versus unbuttressed comparison in this large trial statistically invalid. Fishel and McKenna compared bovine pericardial buttressing with a less expensive bovine collagen material (n=56). Unfortunately, the bovine collagen reinforced patients had an average 2-day longer chest tube duration, which offset any fiscal advantage to the use of the cheaper collagen product.[36]

Within NETT, 9 of the 17 centers performing LVRS participated in a substudy randomizing patients to ePTFE versus bovine pericardium buttressing. No differences in incidence or duration of AL were identified based on the assigned buttress material. Analysis of AL data from the NETT demonstrated that 90% of patients undergoing LVRS experience some degree of AL, with 47% of surgical patients having AL longer than 1 week, and 66 patients (11% of the entire surgical cohort) having a PAL of greater than 30 days duration. Propensity matching within the NETT demonstrated PAL to be associated with an increased risk of mortality, unplanned return to the ICU, pneumonia, and prolonged length of stay.[4] PAL was independent of approach (VATS versus sternotomy), stapler brand, buttress type (bovine pericardium versus ePTFE), or intraoperative adjuncts such as pleural tenting or the use of sclerosants. AL prevalence and duration were associated with patient factors such as the degree of pleural adhesions, the use of inhaled corticosteroids, and declining diffusion capacity.

MANAGEMENT OF PROLONGED AIR LEAK

The management of a PAL is at the core of the art of thoracic surgery. There is little evidence beyond small case series or single case reports to guide the clinician. The typical management protocol should be an orderly progression from watchful waiting to progressively more invasive interventions. Reoperative surgery rarely is required, with large series citing an incidence of less than 2%.[7,9,12]

The use of ambulatory one-way valves—the most commonly used being Heimlich Valves (BD Bard-Parker, Franklin Lakes, New Jersey)—has facilitated earlier hospital discharge for many patients after pulmonary resection.[5] PAL is associated with a higher incidence of other respiratory and cardiac complications,[4] but one-way valves have been used successfully in experienced centers with close outpatient follow-up.[37]

Observation of the ambulatory patient who has a one-way valve in place often reveals little or no AL with tidal breathing but obvious leak with forced exhalation or cough. In the presence of a residual space on chest radiographs, this may signal closure of the parenchymal fistula with a persistent pleural space as the source of the forced AL. In the LVRS emphysema population, empiric removal of such tubes may be risky; however, a trial of provocative clamping as advocated by Kirshner[5,38] can be used to signal safe tube removal.

For patients for whom watchful waiting is unacceptable or for those who cannot progress to water seal or use of a one-way valve, the next incremental invasive step to remedy a PAL would be to instill a pleural sclerosant. The success of pleural sclerosis is predicated on visceral to parietal pleural apposition, which, if absent, may lead to failure of the procedure. Doxycycline or talc[39,40] and autologous blood[41,42] have been found effective sclerosants for selected patients who have PAL after pulmonary resection. The use of autologous blood patches after prolonged chest tube drainage may be associated with higher pleural space infection rates. No systematic evaluation of such agents for PAL after LVRS has been published.

Endoscopic interventions for PAL include the use of metallic coils, fibrin glue,[43] and one-way endobronchial valves originally designed for bronchoscopic lung volume reduction.[44] These applications, however, are no more than successful case reports and underscore the need for individualized clinical decision making when assessing risk and reward. A prospective, compassionate use trial of an endobronchial valve system to salvage spectacular or life-threatening postoperative PAL is ongoing.[45]

Surgical re-exploration to control AL is a rare occurrence. In 580 patients undergoing LVRS in NETT, only 17 (2.9%) required such a drastic intervention.[46] If indicated because of magnitude of the AL or failure of all other conservative measures, the specific reintervention has included restapling, anatomic lobectomy, use of topical sealants[47] or obliteration of the residual space with muscle flaps,[48,49] or omentum.[50]

ACKNOWLEDGMENTS

The authors would like to acknowledge the technical assistance of Donna Minagawa in constructing this article.

REFERENCES

1. Varela G, Jimenez MF, Novoa N, et al. Estimating hospital costs attributable to prolonged air leak in pulmonary lobectomy. Eur J Cardiothorac Surg 2005;27:329–33.
2. Brunelli A, Xiume F, Al Refai M, et al. Air leaks after lobectomy increase the risk of empyema but not of cardiopulmonary complications: a case-matched analysis. Chest 2006;130:1150–6.
3. Cho MH, Malhotra A, Donahue DM, et al. Mechanical ventilation and air leaks after lung biopsy for acute respiratory distress syndrome. Ann Thorac Surg 2006;82:261–6.
4. DeCamp MM, Blackstone EH, Naunheim KS, et al. Patient and surgical factors influencing air leak after lung volume reduction surgery: lessons learned from the National Emphysema Treatment Trial. Ann Thorac Surg 2006;82:197–206.
5. Cerfolio RJ, Bass CS, Pask AH, et al. Predictors and treatment of persistent air leaks. Ann Thorac Surg 2002;73:1727–30.
6. Irshad K, Feldman LS, Chu VF, et al. Causes of increased length of hospitalization on a general thoracic surgery service: a prospective observational study. Can J Surg 2002;45:264–8.
7. Abolhoda A, Liu D, Brooks A, et al. Prolonged air leak following radical upper lobectomy: an analysis of incidence and possible risk factors. Chest 1998; 113:1507–10.
8. Bardell T, Petsikas D. What keeps postpulmonary resection patients in hospital? Can Respir J 2003;10:86–9.
9. Linden PA, Bueno R, Colson YL, et al. Lung resection in patients with preoperative FEV1 <35% predicted. Chest 2005;127:1984–90.
10. Brunelli A, Monteverde M, Borri A, et al. Comparison of water seal and suction after pulmonary lobectomy: a prospective, randomized trial. Ann Thorac Surg 2004;77:1932–7.
11. Cerfolio RJ. Chest tube management after pulmonary resection. Chest Surg Clin N Am 2002;12:507–27.
12. Stolz AJ, Schutzner J, Lischke R, et al. Predictors of prolonged air leak following pulmonary lobectomy. Eur J Cardiothorac Surg 2005;27:334–6.
13. Stolz AJ, Schutzner J, Lischke R, et al. Pulmonary resections and prolonged air leak. Cas Lek Cesk 2005;144:304–7.
14. Wain JC, Kaiser LR, Johnstone DW, et al. Trial of a novel synthetic sealant in preventing air leaks after lung resection. Ann Thorac Surg 2001;71(5):1623–8.
15. Stammberger U, Klepetko W, Stamatis G, et al. Buttressing the staple line in lung volume reduction surgery: a randomized three-center study. Ann Thorac Surg 2000;70(6):1820–5.
16. Hazelrigg SR, Boley TM, Naunheim KS, et al. Effect of bovine pericardial strips on air leak after stapled pulmonary resection. Ann Thorac Surg 1997;63:1573–5.
17. Serra-Mitjans M, Belda-Sanchis J, Rami-Porta R. Surgical sealant for preventing air leaks after pulmonary resections in patients with lung cancer. Cochrane Database Syst Rev 2005;(3):CD003051.
18. Anegg U, Lindenmann J, Matzi V, et al. Efficiency of fleece-bound sealing (TachoSil) of air leaks in lung surgery: a prospective randomised trial. Eur J Cardiothorac Surg 2007;31:198–202.
19. Venuta F, Diso D, De Giacomo T, et al. Use of a polymeric sealant to reduce air leaks after lobectomy. J Thorac Cardiovasc Surg 2006;132(2):422–3.
20. Droghetti A, Schiavini A, Muriana P, et al. A prospective randomized trial comparing completion technique of fissures for lobectomy: stapler versus precision dissection and sealant. J Thorac Cardiovasc Surg 2008;136(2):383–91.
21. Matsumoto I, Ohta Y, Oda M, et al. Free pericardial fat pads can act as sealant for preventing alveolar air leaks. Ann Thorac Surg 2005;80(6):2321–4.

22. Brunelli A, Al Refai M, Monteverde M, et al. Pleural tent after upper lobectomy: a randomized study of efficacy and duration of effect. Ann Thorac Surg 2002;74(6):1958–62.

23. Okur E, Kir A, Halezeroglu S, et al. Pleural tenting following upper lobectomies or bilobectomies of the lung to prevent residual air space and prolonged air leak. Eur J Cardiothorac Surg 2001;20(5):1012–5.

24. Toker A, Dilege S, Tanju S, et al. Perioperative pneumoperitoneum after lobectomy–bilobectomy operations for lung cancer: a prospective study. Thorac Cardiovasc Surg 2003;51(2):93–6.

25. Cerfolio RJ, Holman WL, Katholi CR. Pneumoperitoneum after concomitant resection of the right middle and lower lobes (bilobectomy). Ann Thorac Surg 2000;70(3):942–6.

26. Cooper JD, Patterson GA, Sundaresan RS, et al. Results of 150 consecutive bilateral lung volume reduction procedures in patients with severe emphysema. J Thorac Cardiovasc Surg 1996;112:1319–29.

27. Cooper JD, Patterson GA. Lung-volume reduction surgery for severe emphysema. Chest Surg Clin N Am 1995;5:815–31.

28. Cerfolio RJ, Bass C, Katholi CR. Prospective randomized trial compares suction versus water seal for air leaks. Ann Thorac Surg 2001;71:1613–7.

29. Marshall MB, Deeb ME, Bleier JI, et al. Suction vs water seal after pulmonary resection: a randomized prospective study. Chest 2002;121:831–5.

30. Brunelli A, Sabbatini A, Xiume F, et al. Alternate suction reduces prolonged air leak after pulmonary lobectomy: a randomized comparison versus water seal. Ann Thorac Surg 2005;80:1052–5.

31. Alphonso N, Tan C, Utley M, et al. A prospective randomized controlled trial of suction versus nonsuction to the underwater seal drains following lung resection. Eur J Cardiothorac Surg 2005;27:391–4.

32. Cooper JD, Trulock EP, Triantafillou AN, et al. Bilateral pneumectomy (volume reduction) for chronic obstructive pulmonary disease. J Thorac Cardiovasc Surg 1995;109:106–16.

33. Cooper JD. Technique to reduce air leaks after resection of emphysematous lung. Ann Thorac Surg 1994;57:1038–9.

34. McKenna RJ Jr, Brenner M, Fischel RJ, et al. Patient selection criteria for lung volume reduction surgery. J Thorac Cardiovasc Surg 1997;114:957–67.

35. DeCamp MM Jr. Technical issues and controversies in lung volume reduction surgery. Semin Thorac Cardiovasc Surg 2002;14:391–8.

36. Fischel RJ, McKenna RJ. Bovine pericardium versus bovine collagen to buttress staples for lung reduction operations. Ann Thorac Surg 1998;65:217–9.

37. McKenna RJ, Fischel RJ, Brenner M, et al. Use of the Heimlich valve to shorten hospital stay after lung reduction surgery for emphysema. Ann Thorac Surg 1996;61:1115–7.

38. Kirschner PA. Provocative clamping and removal of chest tubes despite persistent leak. Ann Thorac Surg 1992;53:740–1.

39. Kilic D, Findikcioglu A, Hatipoglu A. A different application method of talc pleurodesis for treatment of persistent air leak. ANZ J Surg 2006;76:754–6.

40. Okereke I, Murthy SC, Alster JM, et al. Characterization and importance of air leak after lobectomy. Ann Thorac Surg 2005;79:1167–73.

41. Shackcloth MJ, Poullis M, Jackson M, et al. Intrapleural instillation of autologous blood in the treatment of prolonged air leak after lobectomy: a prospective randomized controlled trial. Ann Thorac Surg 2006;82:1052–6.

42. Lang-Lazdunski L, Coonar AS. A prospective study of autologous blood patch for persistent air leak after pulmonary resection. Eur J Cardiothorac Surg 2004;26:897–900.

43. Shimizu J, Takizawa M, Yachi T, et al. Postoperative bronchial stump fistula responding well to occlusion with metallic coils and fibrin glue via a tracheostomy. Ann Thorac Cardiovasc Surg 2005;11:104–8.

44. Ferguson JS, Sprenger K, Van Natta T. Closure of a bronchopleural fistula using bronchoscopic placement of an endobronchial valve designed for treatment of emphysema. Chest 2006;129:479–81.

45. Sterman D, Gillespie C, Cerfolio R, et al. Multicenter experience with bronchial valve treatment of life-threatening prolonged air leaks. Eur Respir J 2008; 32:262s–3s.

46. McKenna RJ Jr, Benditt JO, DeCamp M, et al. Safety and efficacy of median sternotomy versus video-assisted thoracic surgery for lung volume reduction surgery. J Thorac Cardiovasc Surg 2004;127: 1350–60.

47. Thistlethwaite PA, Luketich JD, Ferson PF, et al. Ablation of persistent air leaks after thoracic procedures with fibrin sealant. Ann Thorac Surg 1999; 67:575–7.

48. Colwell AS, Mentzer SJ, Vargas SO, et al. The role of muscle flaps in pulmonary aspergillosis. Plast Reconstr Surg 2003;111:1147–50.

49. Francel TJ, Lee GW, Mackinnon SE, et al. Treatment of long-standing thoracostoma and bronchopleural fistula without pulmonary resection in high-risk patients. Plast Reconstr Surg 1997;99:1046–53.

50. Nonami Y, Ogoshi S. Omentopexy for empyema due to lung fistula following lobectomy. A case report. J Cardiovasc Surg (Torino) 1998;39:695–6.

Decision Making in the Management of Secondary Spontaneous Pneumothorax in Patients with Severe Emphysema

K. Robert Shen, MD[a],*, Robert J. Cerfolio, MD[b]

KEYWORDS

- Secondary • Spontaneous • Pneumothorax
- Management • Emphysema

Spontaneous pneumothorax by definition is the development of air in the pleural space between the lung and the chest wall, which occurs without any antecedent trauma or iatrogenic factors. Traditionally, spontaneous pneumothorax is classified further as primary or secondary. Although there are some common features in terms of the presentation, diagnosis, and management, this subclassification recognizes that the two types of spontaneous pneumothorax often are considered and managed as distinct clinical entities. Primary spontaneous pneumothoraces occur in persons without clinically apparent lung disease. Secondary spontaneous pneumothoraces occur in those individuals who have known widespread generalized lung disease causing chronic respiratory symptoms, impaired pulmonary function, and abnormalities on chest imaging. In contrast to the clinical course of a primary spontaneous pneumothorax, which is usually benign, secondary spontaneous pneumothorax can be a potentially life-threatening event because of the patients' associated marginal pulmonary function and often associated limited cardiopulmonary reserve. Chronic obstructive pulmonary disease (COPD) is the most common cause of secondary spontaneous pneumothorax.[1,2]

EPIDEMIOLOGY

The incidence of secondary spontaneous pneumothorax in the general population is similar to that of primary spontaneous pneumothorax (approximately 6.3 cases per 100,000 men per year and 2.0 cases per 100,000 women per year).[3] The incidence of secondary spontaneous pneumothorax in patients who have COPD is significantly higher. It has been estimated to occur in approximately 26 cases per 100,000 patients who have COPD per year.[4] If these figures are extrapolated to the 17.1 million adults in the United States who are estimated to have COPD,[5] one can anticipate approximately 4500 new cases of secondary pneumothorax per year in patients who have COPD.

Most COPD patients who develop spontaneous pneumothorax are older than 50 years of age, and

[a] Department of Surgery, Division of General Thoracic Surgery, Mayo Clinic and Mayo Foundation, 200 First Street, Southwest, Rochester, MN 55905, USA
[b] Department of Surgery, Division of Cardiothoracic Surgery, University of Alabama at Birmingham, 703 19th Street South, ZRB 739, Birmingham, AL 35294, USA
* Corresponding author.
E-mail address: shen.krobert@mayo.edu (K.R. Shen).

Thorac Surg Clin 19 (2009) 233–238
doi:10.1016/j.thorsurg.2009.02.003
1547-4127/09/$ – see front matter © 2009 Elsevier Inc. All rights reserved.

the event is often a marker of the severity of their disease. Patients who have more severe COPD tend to develop spontaneous pneumothoraces more frequently. Patients who have a forced expiratory value in one second (FEV_1) of less than 1 L, or a ratio of FEV_1 to forced vital capacity (FVC) of less than 40%, are at greatest risk. In a Veterans Administration (VA) cooperative study on 171 patients who had a secondary spontaneous pneumothorax, 51 patients (30%) had an FEV_1 less than 1 L, and 56 patients (33%) had an FEV_1/FVC ratio of less than 40%.[6]

PATHOPHYSIOLOGY

The most common cause of secondary spontaneous pneumothorax in patients who have emphysema is the rupture of blebs or bullae. Blebs are well-circumscribed, subpleural air spaces separated from the underlying lung parenchyma by a thin layer of visceral pleura. Blebs are typically small and peripheral, and most are located at the lung apices. Commonly, several blebs will coalesce to form a giant bulla. Bulla are emphysematous spaces larger than 1 cm in diameter in the inflated lung. Bulla result from the destruction of alveolar walls, and they can be associated with any variety of emphysema.

The exact mechanism of bulla formation remains controversial. One commonly accepted hypothesis is that airway inflammation plays a significant role in the pathogenesis. Smoking induces influx of neutrophils and macrophages, which causes degradation of elastic fibers in the lung. This degradation causes an imbalance in the protease–antiprotease and oxidant–antioxidant systems.[7,8] Once bulla have formed in patients who have COPD, airway inflammation or coughing can induce obstruction of the small airways, increasing alveolar pressure. When alveolar pressure exceeds the pressure in the interstitium of the lung, the alveolus can rupture. Air from the ruptured alveolus then moves retrograde along the bronchovascular bundle to the hilum, causing pneumomediastinum. As mediastinal pressure rises, rupture of the mediastinal pleura occurs, resulting in pneumothorax.[9,10] Air from a ruptured alveolus in a subpleural location, such as occurs with blebs, also can move directly into the pleural space as a result of a breach in the visceral pleura.

Accumulating air in the pleural space results in a decrease in vital capacity and an increase in the alveolar–arterial oxygen gradient. Hypoxemia ensues because of increased shunting and a lower ventilation–perfusion ratio. The degree of shunting increases with the size of the pneumothorax. This can result in significant hypercapnea, with $PaCO_2$ often exceeding 50 mm Hg.

CLINICAL PRESENTATION

In patients with moderate-to-severe COPD, the clinical symptoms associated with the development of a spontaneous secondary pneumothorax are much more severe than those associated with primary spontaneous pneumothorax. These symptoms can be life-threatening. Rapidly progressive and alarming degrees of dyspnea usually associated with pleuritic chest pain can develop after a spontaneous pneumothorax in these already marginal patients. The dyspnea frequently can seem out of proportion to the size of the pneumothorax because of the low cardiopulmonary reserve that these patients often have. In one series from the Mayo Clinic concerning 57 patients who had COPD with spontaneous pneumothorax, all patients presented with dyspnea, and 42 (74%) had pleuritic chest pain on the side of the pneumothorax.[4] In addition, five patients were cyanotic, and four patients were hypotensive. In the 18 patients who had arterial blood gases obtained at the time of admission, the mean PaO_2 was 48 mm Hg, and the mean $PaCO_2$ was 58 mm Hg. In the VA cooperative study, the PaO_2 was below 55 mm Hg in 20 of 118 (17%) patients and below 45 mm Hg in 5 of 118 patients (4%). The $PaCO_2$ exceeded 50 mm Hg in 19 of 118 patients (16%) and exceeded 60 mm Hg in 5 of 118 patients (4%).[6]

Secondary spontaneous pneumothorax in patients who have COPD is associated with significant morbidity and mortality. When four older series totaling 174 COPD patients who had spontaneous pneumothorax are combined, the mortality rate was 16%.[4,11–13] Causes of death included sudden death before chest tube insertion, respiratory failure within the first 24 hours, late respiratory failure, and massive gastrointestinal bleeding. In a study of 303 patients who had secondary pneumothorax from Norway, COPD patients had a fourfold increased relative risk of mortality compared with non-COPD patients.[13]

As a result of decreased lung vascularity and diseased lung parenchyma, patients who have COPD and pneumothorax are also more likely to have prolonged air leaks. COPD patients are also more likely to develop pneumonia or an empyema after chest tube placement when compared with non-COPD patients.[13]

DIAGNOSIS

Making a clinical diagnosis of a spontaneous pneumothorax in emphysema patients who already have dyspnea is often difficult. The physical examination findings are often subtle and not as helpful as they are in patients who have primary spontaneous pneumothorax. These patients already have hyperexpanded lungs and distant breath sounds over both lungs. As a result, when a pneumothorax develops, the ability to detect decreased tactile fremitus or hyper-resonant percussion sounds is more difficult than in patients who have normal lungs. The possibility of a spontaneous pneumothorax always should be considered and ruled out in a patient with COPD who develops unexplained dyspnea, particularly if unilateral chest pain is also present. Using chest radiographs to diagnose pneumothorax in patients who have COPD is also less reliable than in patients who have primary spontaneous pneumothorax. The radiographic appearance of the pneumothorax is altered by the loss of elastic recoil of the lung and the presence of air trapping in the diseased lung. In patients who have emphysema and a pneumothorax, normal areas of the lung collapse more completely than diseased areas with large bulla or severe emphysematous changes. Subcutaneous emphysema, which is more common in patients who have severe COPD, also may obscure the pneumothorax. Patients who have bullous emphysema may have radiographic evidence of a large bulla that can be mistaken for a pneumothorax. Alternatively, the presence of a pneumothorax can be overlooked on the initial chest radiograph in patients who have large bulla. One radiographic feature that distinguishes a pneumothorax from bulla is the demonstration of a visceral pleural line. It is sometimes difficult to see this line, because the lung is hyperlucent and there are minimal differences in radio density between the pneumothorax and the emphysematous lung. The pleural line with a pneumothorax runs parallel and usually is oriented in convex fashion toward the lateral chest wall. Bullous lesions that abut the chest wall have a concave appearance. It is important to make the distinction between a large bulla and a pneumothorax, because the latter should be treated with a chest tube. CT of the chest should be performed if there is any doubt as to whether the patient has a pneumothorax or a giant bulla, because the two conditions can be differentiated with this study.[14] Information from CT scans of the chest also can be helpful in selecting the appropriate site for chest tube placement.

In patients who have COPD, occasionally secondary spontaneous pneumothorax can result from high-grade bronchial obstruction, either from mucous plugging or an obstructing primary carcinoma of the lung. This is also an important distinction to make, because these patients should be managed with bronchoscopy rather than tube thoracostomy. When a patient has a collapsed lung, one should look for evidence of air bronchograms in the lung on the chest radiograph. Air bronchograms are absent when there is an endobronchial obstruction, but otherwise they are present.[15]

MANAGEMENT AND TREATMENT OPTIONS

The goals of treatment of the patient with COPD who develops a spontaneous pneumothorax are the same as for those with primary pneumothorax: evacuate air from the pleural space, achieve pleural–pleural apposition, and decrease the likelihood of recurrences. Lack of achievement of these treatment goals, however, has greater sequela in the patient who has a secondary spontaneous pneumothorax. Because the occurrence of a pneumothorax in a patient who has severe emphysema can be life-threatening, a much more aggressive approach is warranted. The treatment options available for the patient who has a secondary pneumothorax are also the same as those for a patient who has a primary spontaneous pneumothorax. Despite a general consensus for more aggressive management of spontaneous pneumothorax in patients who have underlying lung disease, however, there is little consensus regarding specific algorithms of care. In 1993, the British Thoracic Society (BTS) released national guidelines for managing spontaneous pneumothorax after consultation with over 150 British respiratory physicians and thoracic surgeons.[16] The American College of Chest Physicians (ACCP) also released a Delphi Consensus Statement on managing spontaneous pneumothorax in 2001.[17] Both BTS and ACCP guidelines recommend that all patients who have a secondary spontaneous pneumothorax be hospitalized. The ACCP recommends placement of a chest tube with the first episode of a spontaneous pneumothorax and an intervention to prevent recurrences.[17] The BTS management guidelines recommend initial management with manual aspiration of the pneumothorax with a French 16 gauge or larger catheter and syringe. Tube thoracostomy is reserved for cases that have failed simple aspiration.[16] The BTS recommends removal of the chest tube 24 hours after resolution of the air leak and re-expansion of the lung. Pleurodesis and other interventions to prevent recurrences are recommended only for patients who have an unresolved air leak or recurrences in the BTS guidelines.

Simple aspiration of a pneumothorax is less likely to be successful in patients who have underlying lung disease.[18] Tube thoracostomy is also less efficacious in secondary pneumothorax than primary pneumothorax. The mean time to resolve an air leak with a chest tube is also longer in patients who have COPD.[12,13] In approximately 20% of COPD patients who have spontaneous pneumothorax, the lung remains unexpanded, or the air leak persists after 15 days.[12,13,19] The routine use of suction to chest tubes has not been shown to improve the outcome.[20] The ACCP consensus statement recommends that if the lung fails to re-expand with the chest tube on water seal alone, suction be instituted.[17]

COPD patients who have spontaneous pneumothorax are at higher risk for recurrence than those patients who have primary spontaneous pneumothorax. In a study of 303 patients who were treated for spontaneous pneumothorax and followed for a median period of 5.5 years, 24 of the 54 (44%) patients with COPD had recurrences. In the patients without COPD, 96 of 247 (39%) had a recurrence.[13] In 1990, the VA reported a cooperative study on 92 patients with a secondary pneumothorax who were treated with chest tubes without pleurodesis. The recurrence rate was 47%, with a median follow up of 3 years.[6] As a result, it is recommended that in COPD patients who have a pneumothorax, once the lung has expanded, further treatment should be applied, even if it is the first episode, to prevent future recurrences. This is also the recommendation of the ACCP consensus statement, but not the BTS guideline.

The interventions that are available to manage patients who have failed to resolve air leaks or re-expand their lung with tube thoracostomy are the same methods used to prevent recurrences. This includes video-assisted thoracoscopic surgery (VATS), medical thoracoscopy, open limited thoracotomy with pleurectomy, or the instillation of a sclerosing agent through the chest tube. The ACCP recommends medical thoracoscopy or VATS as the preferred technique, with a muscle-sparing (axillary) thoracotomy as an alternative.[17] The BTS recommends open thoracotomy, with VATS reserved only for those patients who cannot tolerate an open procedure.[21] These heterogeneous recommendations highlight the fact that there are limited data comparing the relative benefit of the various interventions, and a dearth of randomized controlled studies. If VATS is available, the authors believe it is the procedure of choice for patients who have COPD, because it provides wide visualization of the pleural space and resection of bulla and pleurodesis can be performed. In addition,

pleurectomy can be performed easily. The authors prefer the use of pericardial-buttressed stapled lines, because they may help prevent prolonged air leaks and also promote adhesions between the lung and chest wall. Some studies suggest that the duration of hospitalization, the length of time needed for postoperative drainage through a chest tube, and the severity of perioperative and postoperative pain are less with VATS than with limited thoracotomy.[22–24] In one study, 22 patients who had secondary spontaneous pneumothorax caused by COPD with a mean age of 70 and a mean preoperative FEV_1 of 40% of predicted underwent VATS for either persistent air leak (18 patients) or recurrent pneumothorax (four patients).[25] The mean operative time was 57 minutes, and only one patient required postoperative mechanical ventilation. The mean duration of postoperative hospitalization was 9 days, and the mean hospitalization before surgery was 18 days. VATS failed in 4 of the 22 patients (18%) and required reoperation with thoracotomy. Two patients died, both of complications related to their pneumothorax. None of the surviving patients had recurrences. Based on the results of these and other similar studies, the ACCP now recommends that for secondary pneumothorax, if there is a persistent air leak or the lung fails to re-expand after 5 days of management with a chest tube, VATS should be performed.[17] Some authors have gone further and suggested that all patients with secondary spontaneous pneumothorax who are safe operative candidates undergo VATS.[17,26]

Recurrence rates after VATS vary from 2% to 14%.[27,28] This compares with a recurrence rate of 0% to 7% for limited thoracotomy.[29,30] Instillation of sclerosing agents through chest tubes for spontaneous pneumothorax has a reported recurrence rate of 8% to 25%.[6,31] Insufflation of talc with VATS has a recurrence rate of 5% to 9%.[32] In a study of 41 patients with advanced emphysema and spontaneous pneumothorax who underwent medical thoracoscopy under local anesthesia with talc poudrage, the recurrence rate was 5% with a median of 35 months follow-up.[33] The mortality rate was 10% in this study.

An additional important factor that should be considered in patients who have advanced emphysema when one is considering an intervention to prevent recurrent pneumothorax is whether the patient is a potential candidate for lung transplantation. In the past, patients were excluded from lung transplantation if previous pleurodesis was performed ipsilateral to the side of the proposed transplantation because of the risk of life-threatening hemorrhage and increased technical difficulty of the procedure after pleurodesis.

Although most lung transplant centers no longer consider prior pleurodesis to be an absolute contraindication to lung transplantation, if pleurodesis is required, a limited anterior pleurodesis is recommended. Talc poudrage should be used only if other techniques have been unsuccessful.

SUMMARY

In contrast to the benign clinical course of a primary spontaneous pneumothorax, secondary pneumothorax in patients who have severe COPD can be a life-threatening event. COPD patients who develop spontaneous pneumothorax require a more aggressive management of their acute respiratory problem and treatment to prevent recurrences. All patients who have secondary spontaneous pneumothorax should be hospitalized and managed with tube thoracostomy and chest roentgenogram. Patients who have a persistent or large air leak or those who lack parietal-to-visceral pleural apposition should undergo VATS early in their hospital stay. During VATS, the leaking bulla should be resected if it can be located, and if not, the most apical bleb should be resected. In addition, pleurodesis along with pleurectomy should be considered in those patients who are safe operative candidates. These techniques help prevent future pneumothoraces from bleb rupture in the patients who have COPD.

REFERENCES

1. Tanaka F, Itoh M, Esaki H, et al. Secondary spontaneous pneumothorax. Ann Thorac Surg 1993;55(2): 372–6.
2. Weissberg D, Refaely Y. Pneumothorax. Chest 2000; 117:1279–85.
3. Dines DE, Clagett OT, Payne WS. Spontaneous pneumothorax in emphysema. Mayo Clin Proc 1970;45:481–7.
4. Melton LJ, Hepper NCG, Offord KP. Incidence of spontaneous pneumothorax in Olmstead County, Minnesota: 1950 to 1974. Am Rev Respir Dis 1979; 120:1379–82.
5. Stang P, Lydick E, Silberman C, et al. The prevalence of COPD using smoking rates to estimate disease frequency in the general population. Chest 2000;117:354–95.
6. Light RW, O'Hara VS, Moritz TE, et al. Intrapleural tetracycline for the prevention of recurrent spontaneous pneumothorax. JAMA 1990;264:2224–30.
7. Fukuda Y, Haraguchi S, Tanaka S, et al. Pathogenesis of blebs and bullae formation in patients with spontaneous pneumothorax: an ultrastructural and immunohistochemical study. Am J Respir Crit Care Med 1994;149:A1022.
8. Wallaert B, Gressier B, Marquette CH, et al. Inactivation of alpha-1 proteinase inhibitor by alveolar inflammatory cells from smoking patients with or without emphysema. Am Rev Respir Dis 1993;147:1537–43.
9. Macklin MT, Macklin CL. Malignant interstitial emphysema of the lungs and mediastinum as an important occult complication in many respiratory diseases and other conditions: an interpretation of the clinical literature in the light of laboratory experiment. Medicine 1944;23:281–358.
10. Sahn SA, Heffner JE. Spontaneous pneumothorax. N Engl J Med 2000;342(12):868–74.
11. Shields TW, Gilschlager GA. Spontaneous pneumothorax in patients 40 years of age and older. Ann Thorac Surg 1966;2:377–83.
12. George RB, Herbert SJ, Shanes JM, et al. Pneumothorax complicating pulmonary emphysema. JAMA 1975;234:389–93.
13. Videau V, Pillgram-Larsen J, Oyvind E, et al. Spontaneous pneumothorax in COPD: complications, treatment and recurrences. Eur J Respir Dis 1987;71: 365–71.
14. Bourgouin P, Cousineau G, Lemire P, et al. Computed tomography used to exclude pneumothorax in bullous lung disease. J Can Assoc Radiol 1985;36:341–2.
15. Fraser RS, Muller NL, Colman N, et al. Diagnosis of diseases of the chest. 4th edition. Philadelphia: WB Saunders; 2000.
16. Miller AC, Harvey JE. Guidelines for the management of spontaneous pneumothorax. BMJ 1993; 307:114–6.
17. Baumann MH, Strange C, Heffner JE, et al. Management of spontaneous pneumothorax. Chest 2001; 119:590–2.
18. Ng AN, Chan KW, Lee JK. Simple aspiration of pneumothorax. Singapore Med J 1994;35(1):50–2.
19. Schoenenberger RA, Haefeli WE, Weiss P, et al. Timing of invasive procedures in therapy for primary and secondary spontaneous pneumothorax. Arch Surg 1991;126:764–6.
20. So SY, Yu DY. Catheter drainage of spontaneous pneumothorax: suction or no suction, early or late removal? Thorax 1982;37:46–8.
21. Henry M, Arnold T, Harvey J. BTS guidelines for the management of spontaneous pneumothorax. Thorax 2003;58(Suppl 2):ii39–52.
22. Passlick B, Born C, Haussinger K, et al. Efficiency of video-assisted thoracic surgery for primary and secondary spontaneous pneumothorax. Ann Thorac Surg 1998;65:324–7.
23. Kim KH, Kim HK, Han JY, et al. Transaxillary minithoracotomy versus video-assisted thoracic surgery for spontaneous pneumothorax. Ann Thorac Surg 1996;61:1510–2.

24. Dumont P, Diemont F, Massard G, et al. Does a thoracoscopic approach for surgical treatment of spontaneous pneumothorax represent progress? Eur J Cardiothorac Surg 1997;11:27–31.

25. Waller DA, Fortz J, Soni AK, et al. Videothoracoscopic operation for secondary spontaneous pneumothorax. Ann Thorac Surg 1994;57:1612–5.

26. Deslauriers J. The management of spontaneous pneumothorax [editorial]. Can J Surg 1994;37(3):182.

27. Andres B, Lujan J, Robles R, et al. Treatment of primary and secondary spontaneous pneumothorax using videothoracoscopy. Surg Laparosc Endosc 1998;8:108–12.

28. Yim AP, Liu HP. Video assisted thoracoscopic management of primary spontaneous pneumothorax. Surg Laparosc Endosc 1997;7:236–40.

29. Horio H, Nomori H, Fuyuno G, et al. Limited axillary thoracotomy vs video-assisted thoracoscopic surgery for spontaneous pneumothorax. Surg Endosc 1998;12(9):1155–8.

30. Crisci R, Coloni GE. Video-assisted thoracoscopic surgery versus thoracotomy for recurrent spontaneous pneumothorax: a comparison of results and costs. Eur J Cardiothorac Surg 1996;10:556–60.

31. Almind M, Lange P, Viskam K. Spontaneous pneumothorax: comparison of simple drainage, talc pleurodesis, and tetracycline pleurodesis. Thorax 1989;44:627–30.

32. Tschopp M, Brutsche M, Frey JG. Treatment of complicated spontaneous pneumothorax by simple talc pleurodesis under thoracoscopy and local anesthesia. Thorax 1997;52:329–32.

33. Lee P, Yap WS, Pek WY, et al. An audit of medical thoracoscopy and talc poudrage for pneumothorax prevention in advanced COPD. Chest 2004;125:1315–20.

Airway Bypass Treatment of Severe Homogeneous Emphysema: Taking Advantage of Collateral Ventilation

Cliff K. Choong, MBBS, FRACS, FRCS[a,b,c,*],
Paulo F.G. Cardoso, MD, PhD[d],
Gerhard W. Sybrecht, MD[e], Joel D. Cooper, MD[f]

KEYWORDS
- Airway bypass stent • Emphysema
- Collateral ventilation • Paclitaxel

Emphysema is a common problem that affects approximately 3.7 million individuals in the United States and is the fourth leading cause of death.[1,2] The World Health Organization estimates that 210 million people worldwide suffer from the disease, and that it led to more than 3 million deaths globally in 2005 (5% of all deaths).[2] Emphysema is anatomically defined as an irreversible increase in the size of the air spaces distal to the terminal bronchials.[1] This increase in size results from the destructive activity of neutrophil and macrophage elastase. The loss of lung tissue alters the physical properties of the lung, leading to a loss of lung elastic recoil and to progressive dynamic hyperinflation of the lungs. The progressive loss of elastic recoil traps the patient in a state of hyperinflation in which forced effort cannot reduce the residual volume because the force exerted to empty the lungs collapses the small airways and obstructs the outflow of gas. These changes result in progressive hyperinflation of the lungs, an enlargement of the thorax, flattening of the diaphragm, increased work of breathing, and reduced exercise tolerance.[3,4] Progressive hyperinflation of the lungs and hyperexpansion of the chest wall also diminishes inspiratory capacity. To maintain adequate minute ventilation the respiratory rate must increase, resulting in an increase in the work of breathing and in dyspnea.

Current medical treatment of emphysema is generally limited to palliative measures that include supplemental oxygen, bronchodilators, anti-inflammatory drugs, and pulmonary rehabilitation. Surgical options in the treatment of emphysema include lung transplantation and lung volume reduction surgery. Both treatment

a Papworth Hospital NHS Foundation Trust, Cambridge, UK
b Department of Surgery, The University of Cambridge, Cambridge, UK
c Department of Surgery, Monash University, Block E, Level 5, Monash Medical Centre, 246 Clayton Road, Clayton, Melbourne, Victoria 3168, Australia
d Department of Surgery, Division of Thoracic Surgery, Santa Casa de Porto Alegre-Pavilhao Pereira Filho Hospital, Universidade Federal de Ciencias da Saude, Porto Alegre, RS, Brazil
e Klinik fur Innere Medizin, Pneumologie, Allergologie, Beatmungs und Umweltmedizi, Meizinische Universitatsklinik, Saarland, Germany
f Division of Thoracic Surgery, University of Pennsylvania Health System, Philadelphia, USA
* Corresponding author. Department of Surgery (MMC), Monash University, Block E, Level 5, Monash Medical Centre, 246 Clayton Road, Clayton, Victoria 3168, Australia.
E-mail address: cliffchoong@hotmail.com (C.K. Choong).

Thorac Surg Clin 19 (2009) 239–245
doi:10.1016/j.thorsurg.2009.04.003
1547-4127/09/$ – see front matter © 2009 Elsevier Inc. All rights reserved.

modalities have specific indications, and their use is limited to selected patients. Lung transplantation can only be performed in a highly selected group of patients and is limited by a lack of donors, the requirement for lifelong immunosuppression therapy, and the permanent risk for rejection and bronchiolitis obliterans. A small subset of patients who have a heterogeneous pattern of emphysema may benefit from lung volume reduction, which has been shown to improve exercise tolerance, the quality of life, and life expectancy.[5]

Airway bypass is the creation of noncollapsing, extra-anatomic passages that connect lung parenchyma to large airways.[6–11] It takes advantage of the increased collateral ventilation in patients who have emphysema to bypass collapsing and obstructed small airways, thereby allowing trapped gas to escape and reduce hyperinflation.[6,7] Collateral ventilation is the ability of gas to move from one part of the lung to another through nonanatomic pathways.[12–15] This phenomenon has been demonstrated to be greatly increased in emphysema, because of the extensive breakdown of alveolar walls and lobular septae.[14,15] Airway bypass is a minimally invasive treatment with the potential to improve pulmonary function and reduce dyspnea in patients who have homogeneous emphysema and potentially could provide meaningful clinical benefit.[6–11] In airway bypass, transbronchial passages are created between segmental or subsegmental bronchi and adjacent lung parenchyma, and these are reinforced with a paclitaxel drug-eluting stent (Exhale Drug-Eluting Stent, Broncus Technologies, Inc., Moutain View, California).[9,11] The purpose of the drug component of the stent is to prevent occlusion of the stented transbronchial passages.[9] This article provides an overview of airway bypass, outlining its concept, development, and experimental studies, and briefly describes the current multicenter prospective randomized double-blind trial evaluating airway bypass, the Exhale Airway Stents for Emphysema (EASE) trial.

CONCEPT AND EVALUATION OF AIRWAY BYPASS

Airway bypass is the creation of transbronchial passages through the bronchial wall at the segmental or subsegmental level (ie, the creation of extra-anatomic bronchopulmonary passages); the passages are supported with self-expanding stents. The airway bypass stent therefore connects lung parenchyma to large airways.[6–11] It takes advantage of the increased collateral ventilation in patients who have emphysema to bypass collapsing and obstructed small airways, thereby allowing trapped gas to escape and

reduce hyperinflation.[6,7] The concept of airway bypass was assessed in two separate experimental studies. The first study conducted was to test the hypothesis that airway bypass could improve pulmonary function in emphysematous lungs by improving expiratory flow and reducing dynamic hyperinflation.[6] Twelve human emphysematous lungs, which were removed at the time of lung transplantation, were placed in an airtight ventilation chamber with the bronchus attached to a tube traversing the chamber wall, and attached to a pneumotachometer.[6] The chamber was evacuated to -10 cm H_2O pressure for lung inflation. A forced expiratory maneuver was simulated by rapidly pressurizing the chamber to 20 cm H_2O while the expiratory flow and volume were continuously recorded. Following baseline measurements, a flexible bronchoscope was then inserted into the airway and a radiofrequency catheter (Broncus Technologies, Inc., Mountain View, California) was used to create a passage through the wall of three separate segmental bronchi into the adjacent lung parenchyma. An expandable stent, 1.5 cm in length and 3 mm in diameter, was then inserted through each passage. Expiratory volumes were then remeasured as described previously. The mean forced expiratory volume in 1 second (FEV_1) increased from 245 mL at baseline to 447 mL, or 83%, following the placement of three bronchopulmonary stents, and the 5-second expired volume increased from 637 mL to 1200 mL or 88%. In 6 of the 12 lungs, two additional stents were then inserted, to make a total of five stents, and forced expiratory measurements again determined. The FEV_1 in the explanted lungs increased by 101% after three stents and by 155% above baseline with the five stents. The study therefore found that airway bypass is a potential therapeutic option for patients who have emphysema with marked hyperinflation and severe homogeneous pulmonary destruction.[6]

The second study undertaken was to evaluate the mechanisms by which airway bypass improves the mechanical properties of the emphysematous lung.[7] The study used 10 emphysematous lungs that were removed during lung transplantations. Lung compartment, mechanic, flow, and volume measurements were determined before and after placement of three or four airway bypass stents. The study found that following airway bypass there was a marked decrease in flow resistance, a significant increase in the maximal expiratory flows and volumes, and the volume after passive deflation decreased by a mean of 1.54 L or 60%. The vital capacity increased by 1.30 L or 132% following the airway bypass procedure. The data show that airway bypass improves the mechanics of breathing in severely emphysematous lungs in vitro and provides strong empiric support that the procedure can improve ventilatory function in patients by reducing flow resistance and gas trapping.[7]

LABORATORY STUDIES EVALUATING THE SAFETY AND FEASIBILITY OF AIRWAY BYPASS

Following a proof of concept that airway bypass improved lung mechanics, expiratory flow, and volume, and reduced trapped gas in explanted emphysematous lungs, the next step was to assess the feasibility and safety of in vivo airway bypass stent placement.[8] A canine model was chosen for the in vivo study because the airway anatomy and size of the study dogs resemble those of humans. With the dogs under general anesthesia, suitable segmental and subsegmental bronchial wall sites were selected by direct visualization with a flexible bronchoscope. Peribronchial blood vessel injury was avoided by using a Doppler probe (Broncus Technologies, Inc.) to detect and avoid areas with peribronchial blood flow. In this study, the airway bypass transbronchial fenestration was formed with a 22-gauge transbronchial needle, and the passage was then dilated with a 2.5-mm angioplasty balloon. A balloon-expandable stainless-steel stent (3 mm long × 3 mm wide) with a sleeve of silicone covering (Broncus Technologies, Inc.) was placed within the fenestration. Seventy stents were placed in 12 dogs.[8] The animals were then bronchoscoped weekly to assess stent patency. The study also set out to assess the influence of topical mitomycin C on the prolongation of stent patency. Out of the 70 stents, 35 served as controls and the other 35 received transbronchoscopic topical application of mitomycin C once weekly to evaluate the effect on the maintenance of stent patency. The mitomycin C stents were divided into four groups according to the number of treatments: group A, 1 treatment only; group B, 4 weeks; group C, 7 weeks; and group D, 9 weeks. Each once-weekly mitomycin C application consisted of 0.2 mL at a concentration of 1 mg/mL, delivered through a small polyethylene catheter. Each dog had both control and mitomycin C stents so that each dog served as its own control. Out of the 70 stents placed, there were four instances of minor and brief bleeding that occurred during stent placement and resolved without incident. One pneumothorax occurred peri-procedurally and was treated by chest tube placement, without any adverse sequelae. There was no mortality associated with the stent placement, and no delayed hemorrhage or pneumothorax occurred.[8] All the control stents were occluded at the 1-week follow-up. The median durations of stent patency for group A (n = 8), group B (n = 9), group C (n = 10), and group D (n = 8) were 3, 8, 13, and greater than 20 weeks, respectively. The study therefore found that airway bypass stent placement can be performed safely in the animal model; however, most stents became occluded within 1 week, but topical mitomycin application resulted in significant prolongation of stent patency.[8]

This study showed that it was feasible and safe to perform airway bypass stent placement in vivo.[8] The control stents were occluded at 1-week follow-up, however, because of reactive inflammatory and granulation processes. The weekly topical applications of mitomycin C inhibited the inflammatory and granulation processes and maintained stent patency. In the consideration of treating patients who have severe emphysema, it is not practical to subject such patients to weekly bronchoscopy and topical application of mitomycin C. A study evaluating paclitaxel-eluting airway bypass stents was therefore undertaken.[9] Paclitaxel has been successfully applied to the prevention of coronary artery restenosis and works by inhibiting mitosis and preventing neointimal proliferation while allowing healing and endothelialisation.[16,17] In the prevention of coronary artery in-stent stenosis, paclitaxel is considered to be best delivered locally on a DES to achieve therapeutic concentrations without the risk for systemic toxicity. On the basis of these findings, another procedural study assessed the potential effect of paclitaxel-eluting stents on airway bypass stent patency.[9] It was hoped that a positive outcome of prolonged stent patency in the animal mode would provide a more practical therapeutic approach for patients who have emphysema.[9] A canine model was again chosen for this study. With the subject dogs under general anesthesia, suitable segmental and subsegmental bronchial wall sites were selected by direct visualization with a flexible bronchoscope. A Doppler probe was then used to detect and avoid sites with adjacent blood vessels. Transbronchial passages were formed with a 25-gauge transbronchial needle-tipped catheter and dilated with a 2.5-mm balloon integrated into the needle catheter (Broncus Technologies, Inc.). A specifically designed expandable stainless steel stent (3 mm long × 3 mm wide) coated with silicone was placed within the passage and expanded until secured in the bronchial wall. Fifty control stents (no paclitaxel impregnation) and 107 paclitaxel-eluting stents were placed in 25 dogs. Each dog had both control and paclitaxel-eluting stents so that each dog served as its own control. The animals underwent bronchoscopy at intervals to assess stent patency. There were eight instances of minor and brief bleeding that occurred during stent placement and all resolved without incident. There was no pneumothorax or death associated with the stent placement. There was no delayed complication, and no identifiable paclitaxel-related toxicity was observed. At 1, 4, 8, and 12 weeks, the patency rates were 10%, 0%, 0%, and 0% for the control stents and 100%, 96%, 76%, and 65% for the paclitaxel stents. The study found that in the animal model, the use of specifically designed paclitaxel-eluting airway bypass stents was both feasible and safe, and these stents resulted in a significant prolongation of stent patency.[9] Based on these findings, the airway bypass paclitaxel-eluting stents were subsequently used for clinical studies.

CLINICAL STUDY EVALUATING THE SAFETY AND FEASIBILITY OF AIRWAY BYPASS

Having shown that airway bypass stent placement was feasible and safe in animal studies, it was also important to assess the feasibility and safety of airway bypass in human subjects. A critical step in the safe performance of this procedure is to create passages through the airway wall into lung parenchyma while avoiding injury to adjacent blood vessels.[10] This clinical study consisted of selection of a target site bronchoscopically, the use of a Doppler catheter to detect and avoid peribronchial blood vessels, and the creation of a passage through the airway wall with a cautery probe.[10] To evaluate the safety of airway bypass, 10 patients were treated during lobectomies for neoplasm. The procedure was done after thoracotomy and immediately before resection and was confined to airways in the lung identified for removal. Airway bypass was also performed in 5 patients undergoing lung transplantation for emphysema just before lung excision to evaluate the procedure in patients who had emphysema. Twenty-nine passages (1–5 per subject) were created in the patients undergoing lobectomy and 18 passages were created (3–4 per subject) in the patients undergoing transplantation. There were two instances of mild bleeding in the patients undergoing lobectomy and no bleeding in the patients undergoing transplantation. Both instances were treated with suction and topical application of epinephrine and resolved without incident. The results of this study confirmed that airway bypass passages can be made safely through the airways of human subjects and these clinical results support further

investigation of the efficacy of the airway bypass procedure in patients who have emphysema.[10]

CLINICAL APPLICATION OF AIRWAY BYPASS WITH PACLITAXEL-ELUTING STENTS: EARLY RESULTS

Following the demonstration of the proof of concept, and the feasibility and safety data in animal and human studies, the next important step was to assess the safety and early clinical results of airway bypass with paclitaxel-eluting stents for selected patients who had severe emphysema.[11] In a multicenter study the airway bypass was performed with a fiberoptic bronchoscope in three steps: identification of a blood vessel–free location with a Doppler probe at the level of segmental bronchi, fenestration of the bronchial wall, and placement of a paclitaxel-eluting stent to expand and maintain the new passage between the airway and adjacent lung tissue.[11] All the adverse events were recorded, along with 1- and 6-month pulmonary function tests and dyspnea index. A total of 35 subjects at 7 centers completed the airway bypass procedure between July 2004 and October 2005. There were 19 men and 16 women with ages between 45 and 81 years (average 62 years). Most subjects (33 of 35, 94%) had homogeneous emphysema. A total of 264 stents were implanted successfully with a median of 8 stents per subject and a range of 2 to 12 stents. Three additional subjects were selected for but did not complete the procedure. One subject did not have stents implanted because of the abundance of blood vessels adjacent to the airway walls as detected by Doppler. In another subject the thickness of the airways prevented stents from being implanted. One death occurred after intraoperative bleeding during treatment (2.6% of all subjects; 0.4% of all passages made). This triggered the safety stopping rules for the study, which resumed after an extensive Data and Safety Monitoring Board investigation. The investigation resulted in several procedural modifications, including the use of bronchus-blocking balloon and the addition of a second Doppler probe-scanning step after bronchial wall fenestration. At 1-month follow-up, statistically significant differences and improvements in residual volume (RV), total lung capacity (TLC), forced vital capacity (FVC), forced expiratory volume, modified Medical Research Council Dyspnea scale (mMRC), 6-minute walk (6MW), and St George's Respiratory Questionnaire were observed. At the 6-month follow-up, there was still significant improvement in residual volume (−400 mL) and dyspnea (−0.5).

The subjects were also divided into two groups based on whether their baseline RV/TLC ratio was above or below the median (0.67) for the entire cohort.[10] In subjects who had baseline RV/TLC above the median, RV was reduced by 1040 mL (−16.2%) at 1 month and 870 mL (−14%) at 6 months. In addition, at 6 months FVC improved by 17% from baseline, which, although not statistically significant, is higher than the 12% improvement that has been identified as clinically significant. For subjects who had RV/TLC at and below the median, RV (−400 mL), FVC (11.1%), and 6MW (28.6 m) had a statistically significant improvement at 1 month, but none of the benefits were maintained at 6 months, with most parameters returning to near or below baseline. This retrospective analysis revealed that the degree of pretreatment hyperinflation may be an important indicator of which patients achieve the best short- and long-term results. It appeared that the severely hyperinflated patients who had baseline RV/TLC of equal to or more than 0.67 experienced better and longer benefits. Overall, the study found that airway bypass procedure reduced hyperinflation and improves pulmonary function and dyspnea in selected patients who have severe emphysema. The duration of benefit appeared to correlate with the degree of pretreatment hyperinflation.[11] These preliminary clinical results supported further evaluation of the procedure and led to a prospective multicenter double-blind study, the Exhale Airway Stents for Emphysema (EASE) Trial.[18]

THE EXHALE AIRWAY STENTS FOR EMPHYSEMA TRIAL

The EASE Trial sets out to evaluate airway bypass and is a multicenter, prospective, randomized, sham-controlled, double-blind study.[18] It is presently ongoing, though enrollment has been completed. The trial is being undertaken by Broncus Technologies, Inc.[18] Broncus is a medical technology company focused on developing minimally invasive medical devices for emphysema and other lung diseases. The company has patented the airway bypass using Exhale Drug-Eluting Stents (DES) and is investigating to determine if airway bypass can provide the first minimally invasive treatment option for homogeneous emphysema. The study aims to evaluate the safety and effectiveness of the Exhale DES to improve pulmonary function and breathlessness in subjects who have homogeneous emphysema with severe hyperinflation. In this multicenter study, approximately 45 centers will enroll from 225 to 450 subjects, randomized 2:1, Exhale DES to sham. The endpoints for safety and effectiveness will be measured at 6 months. All subjects will receive standard medical management and safety assessment throughout 12 months of participation. Treated subjects will be examined and evaluated annually for 4 additional years following 12 months of safety assessment. The study uses a Bayesian study design. These 45-subject increment looks continue until accrual is stopped or 450 subjects are accrued.

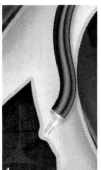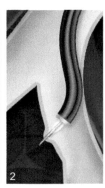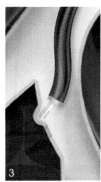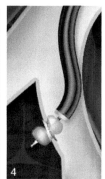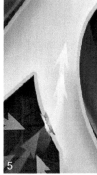

Fig. 1. Steps in airway bypass procedure. The steps involved are: **(1)** Suitable segmental bronchial wall site is selected by direct visualization with a flexible bronchoscope. A Doppler probe is then used to detect and avoid sites with peribronchial blood vessels. **(2)** A transbronchial passage is then formed with a 25-gauge transbronchial needle-tipped catheter and dilated with a 2.5-mm balloon integrated into the needle catheter. **(3)** The Doppler catheter is again used to recheck and ensure the area is absent of peribronchial blood vessels before stent placement. **(4)** The paclitaxel-eluting airway bypass stent is positioned and expanded until secured about the bronchial wall. **(5)** The airway bypass stent forms a new extra-anatomic bronchopulmonary passage and allows trapped gas to escape.

All serious adverse events (SAEs) will be solicited, reported, followed to resolution, and adjudicated. The primary safety endpoint is a comparison of a composite of five SAEs endpoint between the treatment and control groups. In the analysis, there are two primary efficacy outcomes, FVC and mMRC, which are combined in a responder analysis. A subject is a success (responder) if their FVC improves by at least 12% of their baseline value and their mMRC improves (is reduced) by at least 1 point at their 6-month follow-up visit. For superior efficacy to be claimed, the probability of a subject being a responder in the treatment arm must be greater than the control arm. The primary efficacy analysis will be on an intent-to-treat basis on all subjects who enter the procedure room for intervention. Secondary endpoints will be analyzed using Bayesian methods and the secondary endpoint RV/TLC ratio will be analyzed for superiority. This secondary endpoint is the only one that will be analyzed for superiority so no adjustment for multiplicities will be made. The following secondary endpoints will be analyzed for informational purposes: RV, FVC, mMRC, FEV_1, St. George's Respiratory Questionnaire, 6MW, and Cycle Ergometry. The number of stents placed will be determined by the investigator's assessment of the anatomic features of the airways and CT data. Stent placement is targeted to segmental airways leading to regions with the highest RV. Up to six DES (optimally a minimum of one per treated lobe, maximum two per treated lobe, six overall) will be placed. The steps for the airway bypass procedure are shown in **Fig. 1**. The right middle lobe is not treated in the study. The EASE trial completed subject enrollment in April of 2009 and is currently in the subject follow-up phase.

SUMMARY

Airway bypass is being investigated as a new form of minimally invasive therapy for the treatment of homogeneous emphysema. It is a bronchoscopic catheter-based procedure that creates transbronchial extra-anatomic passages at the bronchial segmental level. The passages are expanded, supported with the expectation that the patency is maintained by paclitaxel drug-eluting airway bypass stents. The concept of airway bypass has been demonstrated in two separate experimental studies.[6,7] These studies have shown that airway bypass takes advantage of collateral ventilation present in homogeneous emphysema to allow trapped gas to escape and reduce hyperinflation. It improves lung mechanics, expiratory flow, and volume. Airway bypass stent placements have been shown to be feasible and safe in both

animal and human studies.[8–10] Paclitaxel-eluting airway bypass stents were found to prolong stent patency and were adopted for clinical studies.[9] A study evaluating the early results of the clinical application of airway bypass with paclitaxel-eluting stents found that airway bypass procedures reduced hyperinflation and improved pulmonary function and dyspnea in selected subjects who have severe emphysema.[11] The duration of benefit appeared to correlate with the degree of pretreatment hyperinflation. These preliminary clinical results supported further evaluation of the procedure and led to the EASE Trial. The EASE Trial is a prospective, multicenter, randomized, double-blind, sham-controlled study. The trial aims to evaluate the safety and effectiveness of the airway bypass to improve pulmonary function and reduce dyspnea in homogeneous emphysema subjects who have severe hyperinflation. The trial is presently ongoing worldwide, though enrollment was completed.

REFERENCES

1. Epidemiology and Statistics Unit, American Lung Association. Trends in COPD (chronic bronchitis and emphysema): morbidity and mortality. April 2009. Available at: http://www.lungusa.org.
2. World Health Organization. Chronic obstructive pulmonary disease. Fact sheet No 315. Geneva (Switzerland): World Health Organization; 2008.
3. Rochester D, Braun N, Arora N. Respiratory muscle strength in chronic obstructive pulmonary disease. Am Rev Respir Dis 1979;119:151–4.
4. Sharp J, Danon J, Druz W, et al. Respiratory muscle function in patients with chronic obstructive pulmonary disease: its relationship to disability and to respiratory therapy. Am Rev Respir Dis 1974;110:154–67.
5. Naunheim KS, Wood DE, Mohsenifar Z, et al. The National Emphysema Treatment Trial Research Group. Long-term follow-up of patients receiving lung-volume-reduction surgery versus medical therapy for severe emphysema by the National Emphysema Treatment Trial Research Group. Ann Thorac Surg 2006;82:431–43.
6. Lausberg HF, Chino K, Patterson GA, et al. Bronchial fenestration improves expiratory flow in emphysematous human lungs. Ann Thorac Surg 2003;75:393–7.
7. Choong CK, Macklem PT, Pierce JA, et al. Airway bypass improves the mechanical properties of explanted emphysematous lungs. Am J Respir Crit Care Med 2008;178:902–5.
8. Choong CK, Haddad FJ, Gee EY, et al. Feasibility and safety of airway bypass stent placement and

influence of topical mitomycin C on stent patency. J Thorac Cardiovasc Surg 2005;129:632–8.

9. Choong CK, Phan L, Massetti P, et al. Prolongation of patency of airway bypass stents with use of drug-eluting stents. J Thorac Cardiovasc Surg 2006;131:60–4.

10. Rendina EA, De Giacomo T, Venuta F, et al. Feasibility and safety of the airway bypass procedure for patients with emphysema. J Thorac Cardiovasc Surg 2003;125:1294–9.

11. Cardoso PFG, Snell GI, Hopkins P, et al. Clinical application of airway bypass with paclitaxel-eluting stents: early results. J Thorac Cardiovasc Surg 2007;134:974–81.

12. Van Allen C, Lindskog G, Richter H. Gaseous interchange between adjacent lung lobules. Yale J Biol Med 1930;2:297–300.

13. Menkes H, Traystman R, Terry P. Collateral ventilation. Fed Proc 1979;38:22–6.

14. Terry PB, Traystman RJ, Newball HH, et al. Collateral ventilation in man. N Engl J Med 1978;298:10–5.

15. Macklem PT. Collateral ventilation. N Engl J Med 1978;298:49–50.

16. Schiff PB, Horwitz SB. Taxol stabilizes microtubules in mouse fibroblast cells. Proc Natl Acad Sci U S A 1980;77:1561–5.

17. Kolodgie FD, John M, Khurana C, et al. Sustained reduction of in-stent neointimal growth with the use of a novel systemic nanoparticle paclitaxel. Circulation 2002;106:1195–8.

18. Exhale Airway Stents for Emphysema (EASE Trial). Available at: http://easetrial.com/. Accessed January 1, 2009.

Treatment of Heterogeneous Emphysema Using the Spiration IBV Valves

Steven C. Springmeyer, MD[a,b],*, Chris T. Bolliger, MD[c,d],
Thomas K. Waddell, MD, Msc, PhD[e], Xavier Gonzalez, MD[a,b],
Douglas E. Wood, MD[f,g]
for the IBV Valve Pilot Trials Research Teams

KEYWORDS

- CT • Emphysema • Lung volume reduction
- Bronchial valve

Lung volume reduction surgery (LVRS) research has demonstrated the best treatment results in patients who have upper lobe (UL)-predominant disease utilizing a bilateral procedure with significant improvements in pulmonary function, exercise capacity, and quality of life.[1] LVRS, however, is associated with significant morbidity and mortality, and a prolonged convalescence, providing an impetus for less invasive techniques to achieve palliation for symptoms of end-stage emphysema. The hypothesis that endoluminal obstruction of airflow into targeted pulmonary segments may result in a similar lung reduction effect led to the development of various endoluminal occlusion efforts to achieve minimally invasive lung reduction. Because LVRS removes approximately one third of each lung, it was postulated that airway-based treatment of three segments of each lung would be similar in effect.

After experiments indicated an airway plug resulted in an unacceptable pneumonia rate in healthy animal lungs, Spiration Incorporated (Redmond, Washington) began development of the IBV valve to block distal airflow without obstructing proximal air and fluid flow. This development work has been summarized[2] and resulted in approval to begin clinical studies in early 2004.

The results with the first 30 subjects treated in this series have been published showing bilateral UL treatment had acceptable safety and significantly improved health-related quality of life (HRQL).[3] It was notable that over 50% of patients responded in their HRQL as measured by the SGRQ, but they did not have a reduction in total lung volume, an improved forced expiratory volume in 1 second (FEV_1), or improved exercise as measured by 6-minute walk distance (6MWT) or cycle ergometry. The authors expanded and extended the study, revised some testing methods, and evaluated other measures of effectiveness.

Doctors Springmeyer and Gonzalez are employees of Spiration Incorporated. Doctors Wood and Bolliger received support for research and consulting fees. Dr. Waddell received support for research.

a School of Medicine, University of Washington, Seattle, WA, USA
b Spiration Incorporated, 6675 185th Avenue Northeast, Redmond, WA 98052, USA
c Department of Medicine, University of Stellenbosch, Cape Town, South Africa
d Tygerberg Hospital, University of Stellenbosch, Clinical Building, 19063, Tygerberg 7505, Cape Town, South Africa
e Toronto General Hospital, 200 Elizabeth Street, EN 10-233, Toronto, Ontario M5G 2C4, Canada
f Department of Thoracic Surgery, University of Washington, Seattle, WA, USA
g University of Washington Medical Center, 1959 Northeast Pacific, AA-115, Box 356310, Seattle, WA 98195 6310, USA
* Corresponding author. Spiration Inc., 6675 185th Avenue NE, Redmond, WA 98052.
E-mail address: sspringmeyer@spiration.com (S.C. Springmeyer).

Thorac Surg Clin 19 (2009) 247–253
doi:10.1016/j.thorsurg.2009.02.005
1547-4127/09/$ – see front matter © 2009 Elsevier Inc. All rights reserved.

Additional clinical sites were added in the United States and internationally. The United States experience is being reported in detail (D. Sterman MD, personal communication, 2008), and the analyses with quantitative CT have been published.[4] Here is summarized the authors' total experience, including international studies.

MATERIALS AND METHODS
Study Population

This case series includes all patients where the intent was bilateral treatment of UL-predominant emphysema. Details on inclusion and exclusion criteria have been published,[3] and these remained consistent throughout the study. In summary, patients who had severe airflow obstruction, hyperinflation, and severe UL predominant emphysema were selected. The National Emphysema Treatment Trial (NETT) method for determination for UL predominance was used.[1]

Patients were on maximal medical management before entering the study. For an improved study design,[5] preprocedure pulmonary rehabilitation was not required, but it was required that subjects walk greater than 140 m in the 6MWT for inclusion.

Procedure

The umbrella shape valves, airway sizing kit, and deployment catheter are used for valve treatment (IBV Valve System, Spiration Inc.). The valves have a nitinol frame with five anchors and six struts as shown in **Fig. 1**. The flexible anchors and struts

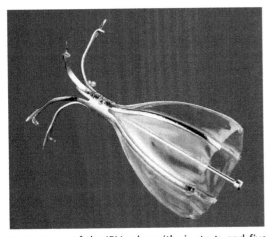

Fig. 1. Image of the IBV valve with six struts and five anchors. Note that the struts are curved inward at the ends to facilitate gliding over the mucosa, and the anchors have pads to control the depth of penetration to about 1 mm into the mucosa. (*Courtesy of* Spiration Incorporated, Redmond, WA; with permission.)

expand radially and conform to tapering, nonoval, or angulated airways. The struts are covered with a thin membrane that prevents distal airflow when held against the airway wall by the struts. The struts are flexible so that air, fluids, or mucus can move past the valve with cough or exhalation, and expand and contract with airway movement during breathing. The valves come in multiple sizes and are compressed into a deployment catheter for delivery to an airway by means of the working channel of a bronchoscope.

The valves are placed into the targeted airways using the deployment catheter and a flexible bronchoscope. Bronchoscopy most often is performed using general anesthesia and endotracheal intubation. Endotracheal intubation is recommended for airway control, use of mechanical ventilation, and when valve removal is anticipated. Anesthesia and ventilation should be sufficient to control cough, reduce airway motion during airway sizing and valve placement, and to prevent forced exhalation with airway narrowing. Details of the procedure and valve deployment have been described previously.[3] The catheter is flexible and allows direct visualization of the desired segment or subsegment while placing valves with the bronchoscope.

Postprocedure and Follow-up

After the procedure, the subjects were observed for 1 night, and then follow-up occurred at 2 weeks and 1 month. For initial subjects, there was a second bronchoscopy after 1 month to observe valves and allow revisions to treatment. This was discontinued after subject 65, because there was no valve migration or erosion in any subject, and the risk of an additional procedure was deemed unnecessary.

Follow-up visits for assessment of adverse events and testing occurred at 3, 6, and 12 months from the initial procedure. These visits included a chest radiograph in all subjects, and in the final 33 subjects, a CT for quantitative analysis (QCT) of regional lung volumes was added at 3 months. The methodology and details regarding quantitative CT are published.[4]

Protocols and Assessments

All sites worked from common protocols, and the data collected were defined prospectively. Standard methods were used for pulmonary function testing. HRQL was assessed using the St. George's Respiratory Questionnaire (SGRQ) with recommended methods and translation where needed. The methods for the 6MWT were within recommended guidelines.[6]

Atelectasis was assessed by reviewing the radiographic reports within 2 weeks of treatment. If atelectasis remained after lung expansion by a chest tube, it was counted as present at the time of pneumothorax.

Adverse events were adjudicated by a clinical events committee, and the trial was supervised by a data safety monitor board. All studies were performed with ethics or institutional review board (IRB) approvals and informed consent.

RESULTS

Ninety-eight subjects were enrolled for bilateral treatment at 13 clinical centers from January 2004 to August 2006. There were 57% males, and the mean age was 65 plus or minus 8 years. Average procedure time for the initial procedure was 58 minutes (range 15 to 187). Valves were placed in segmental airways 74% of the time and 26% in subsegmental airways. Six hundred fifty-nine valves were placed, and all desired airways were treated with the exception of two instances where the catheter could not be passed into the apical segment of the left UL (LUL). Follow-up procedures included revisions with 24 valves replaced and 31 additional valves. Bilateral treatment was done in all but three subjects, where there was a pre-existing contracted UL. The lingular segments of the LUL were not treated except in 18 cases. In one case, the right middle lobe was added to bilateral UL treatment, but not the lingular segments.

There were no instances in any subject of valve migration or expectoration. The absence of migration was confirmed with inspection at follow-up bronchoscopy and chest radiographs. No instances of erosion of the airway by a valve occurred.

Baseline and follow-up results for lung volumes, FEV_1, walking distance, and SGRQ are shown in **Table 1**. The results with the initial 30 subjects[3] were confirmed by the entire cohort of 98 subjects. There were clinically meaningful improvements in HRQL as measured by the SGRQ but not other parameters. Also similar to the initial results, 55.7% of subjects had a 4-point or greater improvement of their SGRQ at 6 months, the clinically meaningful improvement of HRQL. Of note, there was not physiologic volume reduction measured by TLC or RV.

Consistent with PFT-measured TLC; there was no change in total lung volume measured by QCT.[4] There were significant lobar volume changes in the treated UL and untreated lobes (NUL), however. At 6 months, the UL were smaller by a mean of 335 mL ($P<.01$), and 87.5% of subjects had a decrease in volume. The NULs were proportionally larger by a mean of 374 mL ($P < .01$), and 94% of subjects had an increase in NUL volume. Similar and significant changes were present at 1 and 3 months. Because the lobar volume changes were highly correlated and proportional, there was no change in the total lung volumes. Importantly, these interlobar shifts in volume correlate with other measures including HRQL ($P < .01$ for NUL increase and SGRQ improvement).[4]

Adverse Events

Procedure-related adverse events included one serious episode and no deaths. The serious episode has been described;[3] the evening after an uneventful procedure, there was chest pain, respiratory distress, cardiac arrest, myocardial infarction, and a 33-day hospitalization. The most common event after a procedure was bronchospasm, which resolved with a bronchodilator treatment in three cases and several bronchodilator treatments in another two. In two cases, the bronchospasm continued for over 24 to 48 hours, so all valves were removed to eliminate the possibility of a valve contribution. These two episodes resolved and were judged possibly or probably related to the valves.

The most common device-related adverse event was pneumothorax, with eight episodes, two of which were observed without an intervention, and four were considered serious events. Five of the subjects had the onset of pneumothorax during the observation period in the hospital after treatment. One fatal tension pneumothorax occurred during sleep on day 4 after a procedure. This subject was among 18 who had treatment of the lingular segments added to the bilateral treatment. Left-sided pneumothorax occurred in 6 of those 18 subjects. Left-side pneumothorax did not occur after the addition of lingular treatment was discontinued following subject number 65.

Atelectasis is associated with both complications and a greater treatment response. Atelectasis was reported in nine subjects (9.2%) within 2 weeks of valve treatment. In five (56%) of these subjects, there was also pneumothorax, and in four it was reported as lobar atelectasis. **Table 2** shows a significant association between atelectasis and pneumothorax ($P < .01$). **Table 3** shows the results separated into subjects with and without atelectasis after treatment. The results show clinically meaningful improvement at 6 months in lung volumes, FEV_1, and SGRQ in six patients who had atelectasis. The 10-fold larger

Table 1
Lung function, walk distance, and health-related quality of life before and after valve placement (mean ± SD)

	Baseline (N)	1 Month (N)	3 Months (N)	6 Months (N)	12 Months (N)
TLC, L	7.67 ± 1.44 (97)	7.63 ± 1.50 (89)	7.69 ± 1.49 (84)	7.58 ± 1.46 (73)	7.54 ± 1.61 (54)
RV, L	4.84 ± 1.10 (97)	4.87 ± 1.17 (89)	5.03 ± 1.20 (84)	4.87 ± 1.16 (73)	4.72 ± 1.25 (54)
Forced expiratory volume in 1 second, L	0.87 ± 0.25 (98)	0.85 ± 0.25 (89)	0.84 ± 0.26 (84)	0.84 ± 0.29 (74)	0.86 ± 0.33 (55)
6 MWD, feet	1109 ± 318 (98)	1101 ± 329 (86)	1120 ± 341 (81)	1162 ± 345 (72)	1188 ± 310 (51)
SGRQ Total score	57 ± 14(95)	53 ± 14 (86)	53 ± 17 (84)	50 ± 18 (71)	48 ± 17 (56)

group, those without atelectasis, also had clinically meaningful improvement in SGRQ, however, with 52.5% of subjects improved by 4 points or greater. Additionally, the subjects without atelectasis did not have the complications associated with atelectasis.

DISCUSSION

This series of pilot studies with the umbrella-shaped IBV valve showed acceptable safety and risk factors for complications, along with significant effectiveness in over half of the subjects, and a novel mechanism of action. This is the only published experience with bronchial valves where multicenter studies were done prospectively with a common protocol. An equal sized series using the Emphasys valve is a summary of data from selected sites using variable selection criteria and different treatment algorithms.[7] Those investigators concluded that unilateral treatment was best and began using complex software-directed analyses of CT scans to guide patient selection and treatment of a single upper or lower lobe.[8]

The authors found advanced age was a risk factor for procedure complications, and adding treatment of the lingula was a risk factor for left-sided pneumothorax. The authors did not have an upper limit to age in this series. Upon review of the experience, the authors noted that 23% of the advanced age group (aged at least 75 years) had complications after bronchoscopy. This rate is low compared with lung volume reduction surgery,[9] but it may be high for a sham procedure in a randomized controlled trial.

Similar to several published series using early versions of the Emphasys valve,[10–12] episodes of pneumothorax began following the authors' initial experience in 30 subjects.[3] These episodes of pneumothorax started after the authors added treatment to the lingular segments to produce

complete bilateral UL occlusion and occurred in one third of those 18 patients.

The IBV valve investigators had a 99.7% success rate of placing valves in the targeted airways, and there was no migration or expectoration. This technical success compares favorably with the 56.2% rate reported in the VENT study with the Zephyr version of the Emphasys valve.[13] In addition, airway sealing and IBV valve function can be observed easily at the time of placement because of visibility of the treatment location through the valve membrane; a suboptimally positioned valve can be removed and replaced.

An association between atelectasis and pneumothorax after treatment with early versions of the Emphasys valve has been observed,[10] and the authors' results support this association. The authors agree that the mechanism of pneumothorax is likely torsion on tissue adjacent to the treated area.[10,12] Their results indicate that about 50% of the subjects who had atelectasis after valve treatment had pneumothorax. Pneumothorax is a complication that can be serious and fatal in patients who have severe chronic obstructive pulmonary disease (COPD). Fortunately, the incidence of pneumothorax after valve treatment has been low, but current technology cannot predict which patients will have atelectasis or pneumothorax. An association between complete

Table 2
Association of pneumothorax and atelectasis after valve treatment

	Atelectasis	
Pneumothorax	Yes	No
Yes	5	6
No	4	83

Table 3
Pulmonary function and SGRQ changes for subjects at 6 months, with and without atelectasis

	ATX-Yes (N)	ATX-No (N)	Total (N)
TLC change (L)	−0.4 ± 0.7 (6)	−0.1 ± 0.6 (66)	−0.07 ± 0.6 (72)
RV change (L)	−0.7 ± 1.0 (6)	0.1 ± 0.8 (66)	0.0 ± 0.8 (72)
Forced expiratory volume in 1 second change (L)	0.14 ± 0.06 (6)	−0.04 ± 0.16 (68)	−0.02 ± 0.16 (74)
SGRQ change	−15.3 ± 14 (6)	−7.3 ± 16 (64)	−8.0 ± 16 (70)
SGRQ responders	5/6 [83%]	34/64 [53.1%]	39/70 [55.7%]

Abbreviation: ATX, atelectasis.

interlobar fissures as assessed by HRCT and atelectasis with bronchial valve treatment has been reported from the VENT study.[14] Incomplete interlobar fissures are presumed to allow more interlobar collateral ventilation (CV), but this was not found with an ex vivo assessment of lungs with severe emphysema removed for transplantation.[15] In addition, intralobar CV, compared with interlobar CV, may be a greater factor regarding lobar atelectasis, especially when not all airways in a lobe are treated. The absence of intralobar CV is the most likely explanation for the authors' increased pneumothorax rate associated with adding the lingular segments to LUL valve treatment. The authors discontinued treatment of the lingular segments of the LUL with resolution of the increased rate of left-sided pneumothorax.

It had been assumed that lung volume reduction from atelectasis was necessary for a treatment response. This means sufficient atelectasis and volume reduction so there is physiologic improvement in chest wall and respiratory muscle mechanics. An exception would be those patients who respond by improving dynamic hyperinflation.[16] The authors' results indicate that most patients who respond to multi-lobar valve treatment do not have physiologic lung volume reduction. They, however, have a proportional shift of inspired volume from the treated lobe to the untreated lobes, an interlobar shift. This type of response has not been reported previously and may not be significant after valve treatment of a single lobe. Treating a single lobe when the contralateral lobe also has high compliance could allow volume to shift to another very diseased lobe, rather than directing ventilation to less compliant and better functioning lung tissue. That suggests interlobar shift requires bilateral or multilobar treatment in order to redirect the inspired volume to less diseased lung.

The authors found this interlobar shift of inspired ventilation with QCT imaging and analyses. This shift of ventilation often is accompanied by a decrease in the density of blood in the UL as measured by QCT, which suggests there is better ventilation and perfusion matching in the NUL.[4] An interlobar volume shift of 350 mL may seem small when considering a static measurement of lung volumes. This 350 mL, however, will be a large fraction of each inspired breath, because a typical resting tidal volume is 500 mL, and patients who have severe emphysema are not able to greatly increase their tidal volume like a healthy person during activity.

Collateral ventilation is most likely both friend and foe for bronchial valve treatment.[17] CV is a friend regarding safety of the procedure by preventing lobar atelectasis with pneumothorax, but a foe regarding effectiveness if it were to eliminate a treatment response. There are likely various degrees of CV in the 98 subjects in the authors' series, even though they were heterogeneous and UL predominant.[18] If low or absent CV resulted in lobar atelectasis, this occurred in about 10% of the authors' subjects. If very high CV prevented any treatment response, this occurred in about 10% of the authors' subjects. The treatment response estimate is based on QCT, where about 90% of subjects have changes in lobar volumes after bilateral IBV valve treatment. Therefore, CV is likely not the bane of bilateral bronchoscopic treatment of emphysema.[19] When there is knowledge of the degree of CV in an individual patient, however, this may guide a tailored treatment plan with safer and more effective treatment.

With current knowledge, a treatment algorithm that enhances an interlobar shift without complete lobar atelectasis is desirable. Such an algorithm should be used until there is a proven method for predicting which patients are at higher risk of atelectasis or pneumothorax. This is being done in the Spiration randomized, controlled trials in the European Union and United States.

In summary, a study of IBV valve treatment of bilateral ULs, performed in international centers by many investigators, demonstrated a very high treatment response, a high responder rate as assessed by health-related quality of life, with an acceptable safety profile. The authors also found that the most common mechanism of action is an interlobar shift of inspired ventilation and not physiologic lung volume reduction.

NOTE

The IBV Valve System has been approved by the Food and Drug Administration as a humanitarian device for use in the control of prolonged air leaks of the lung, or significant air leaks that are likely to become prolonged air leaks following lobectomy, segmentectomy and LVRS. The effectiveness for this use has not been demonstrated. Please see the *Instructions for Use* available at http://www.fda.gov/cdrh/ode/H060002sum.html, or contact Spiration Inc. for further information. The IBV Valve System has received market clearance through CE Mark for the treatment of diseased and damaged lung, a broad indication that includes the treatment of emphysema and the resolution of air leaks.

IBV VAVLE PILOT TRIALS RESEARCH TEAMS

Cedars Medical Center, Los Angeles: Robert McKenna, MD (principal investigator); Zab Mohsenifar, MD (coprincipal investigator); Carol Geaga, RN (principal clinic coordinator); Cleveland Clinic Foundation (CCF), Cleveland, Ohio: Atul Mehta, MD (principal investigator); Thomas Gildea, MD (coprincipal investigator); Yvonne Meli, RN (principal clinic coordinator); Michael Machuzak, MD; Sudish Murthy, MD; Columbia University Medical Center New York: Roger Maxfield, MD (principal investigator); Mark Ginsburg, MD (coprincipal investigator); Fran Brogan (principal clinic coordinator); Angela Di Mango, MD; Bryon Thomahow, MD; Chun Yip, MD; Joshua Sonett, MD; Patricia Jellen, RN; Duke University Medical Center, Durham, North Carolina: Momen Wahidi, MD (principal investigator); Thomas D'Amico, MD (coprincipal investigator); Linda S. Brown (principal clinic coordinator); John Davies, MA, RRT; Indiana University Hospital, Indianapolis: Praveen Mathur, MD (principal investigator); Francis Sheski, MD (coprincipal investigator); Kathleen Keller, RN (principal clinic coordinator); Annette Hempfling, RN; North Shore–Long Island Jewish Health System, Manhasset, NY: David Ost, MD (principal investigator); Talwar Arunabh, MD (coprincipal investigator); Romona Ramdeo, RN (principal clinic coordinator); Shirley Lilavois, RN; Ohio State University, Columbus, OH: Philip Diaz, MD (principal investigator); Patrick Ross, MD (coprincipal investigator); Mahasti Rittinger, RCP, RRT (principal clinic coordinator) Abbas El-Sayed Abbas, MD; Bonnie Massey; Janice Drake, CRTT,

CCRP; Maria Lucarelli, MD; Nitin Bhatt, MD; Rachael Compton; Shaheen Islam, MD; Toronto General Hospital, Toronto, Ontario, Canada: Thomas Waddell, MD, MSc, PhD, FRCSC (principal investigator); Marc de Perrot, MD (coprincipal investigator); Milan Patel, MD, FRCP (coprincipal investigator); Jennifer Hornby (principal clinic coordinator); Debbie Murnaghan; Tygerberg Hospital, University of Stellenbosch, Cape Town, South Africa: Chris Bolliger, MD (principal investigator); Margaret Pontiac (principal clinical coordinator); University of Alabama at Birmingham, Birmingham, Alabama: Robert Cerfolio, MD, (principal investigator); Sara Pereira, MD, (coprincipal investigator); Jeana Alexander, RN, BSN, (principal clinic coordinator); Ayesha Bryant; Chad Miller, MD; Keith Willie, MD; Sandra Calloway; University of Pennsylvania Medical Center, Philadelphia: Daniel Sterman, MD (principal investigator); Ali Musani, MD (coprincipal investigator); Barbara Finkel, MSN, RN, CCRC (principal clinic coordinator); Andrew Haas, MD; Colin Gillespie, MD; David Lipson, MD Michael Machuzak, MD; Michael Sims, MD; Steven Leh, MD; University of Virginia Health System, Charlottesville, VA: Jonathon Truwit, MD (principal investigator); Yun Michael Shim, MD (Coprincipal investigator); Peggie Donowitz, RN (principal clinic coordinator); Ajeet Vinayak, MD; Halim Hanna, MD; Monojkumar Patel, MBBS; Renee Campbell, RN; University of Washington Medical Center, Seattle, Washington: Douglas Wood, MD (principal investigator); Michael Mulligan, MD (coprincipal investigator); Jo Ann Broeckel Elrod PhD (principal clinic coordinator); Linda Harrison, CCRC. The authors also wish to thank the University of British Columbia for CT review and quantitative analyses, Harvey O. Coxson, PhD, Paola V. Nasute Fauerbach, MD, Claudine Storness-Bliss, Sebastian Cogswell, Nestor L. Müller, MD, PhD.

REFERENCES

1. National Emphysema Treatment Trial Research Group. A randomized trial comparing lung volume reduction with medical therapy for severe emphysema. N Engl J Med 2003;348:2059–73.
2. Springmeyer SC, Wood DE. Development of a bronchial valve for treatment of severe emphysema. Available at: http://www.ctsnet.org/portals/thoracic/newtechnology.
3. Wood DE, McKenna RJ Jr, Yusen RD, et al. A multicenter trial of an intrabronchial valve for treatment of severe emphysema. J Thorac Cardiovasc Surg 2007;133(1):65–73, 3.
4. Coxson HO, Nasute Fauerbach PV, Storness-Bliss C, et al. The computed tomography

assessment of lung volume changes after bronchial valve treatment. Eur Respir J 2008;32:1443–50.

5. Springmeyer SC, Casaburi R, Make B, et al. Pulmonary rehabilitation and clinical trial design in patients with severe COPD. COPD 2008;5:305–9.

6. American Thoracic Society. ATS statement: guidelines for the six-minute walk test. Am J Respir Crit Care Med 2002;166:111–7.

7. Wan IYP, Toma TP, Geddes DM, et al. Bronchoscopic lung volume reduction for end-stage emphysema. Chest 2006;129:518–26.

8. Strange C, Herth FJF, Kovitz KL, et al. Design of the endobronchial valve for emphysema palliation trial (VENT): a nonsurgical method of lung volume reduction. BMC Pulm Med 2007;7:10.

9. Naunheim KS, Wood DE, Krasna MJ, et al. Predictors of operative mortality and cardiopulmonary morbidity in the National Emphysema Treatment Trial. J Thorac Cardiovasc Surg 2006;131(1):43–53.

10. Toma TP, Hopkinson NS, Hillier J, et al. Bronchoscopic volume reduction with valve implants in patients with severe emphysema. Lancet 2003; 361(9361):931–3.

11. Yim AP, Hwong TM, Lee TW, et al. Early results of endoscopic lung volume reduction for emphysema. J Thorac Cardiovasc Surg 2004;127:1564–73.

12. Venuta F, Giacomo TD, Rendina EA, et al. Bronchoscopic lung-volume reduction with one-way valves in patients with heterogenous emphysema. Ann Thorac Surg 2005;79:411–6 [discussion: 416–7].

13. Ernst A, Herth FJ, McLennan G, et al. Contribution of technical success of valve placement to functional outcome in endobronchial lung volume reduction. Am J Respir Crit Care Med 2008;177: A829.

14. Abtin F, Goldin JG, Strange C, et al. The influence of fissural anatomy on the treatment outcome of patients with emphysema. Am J Respir Crit Care Med 2008;177:A755.

15. Higuchi T, Reed A, Oto T, et al. Relation of interlobar collaterals to radiological heterogeneity in severe emphysema. Thorax 2006;61:409–13.

16. Hopkinson NS, Toma TP, Hansell DM, et al. Effect of bronchoscopic lung volume reduction on dynamic hyperinflation and exercise in emphysema. Am J Respir Crit Care Med 2005;171(5):453–60.

17. Noppen M. Collateral ventilation in end-stage emphysema: a blessing or a curse for a new bronchoscopic treatment approaches (or both)? Respiration 2007;74:493–5.

18. Cetti EJ, Moore AJ, Geddes DM. Collateral ventilation. Thorax 2006;61:371–3.

19. Fessler HE. Collateral ventilation, the bane of bronchoscopic volume reduction. Am J Respir Crit Care Med 2005;171:423–5.

Endobronchial Treatment of Emphysema with One-Way Valves

Federico Venuta, MD[a],*, Erino A. Rendina, MD[b],
Giorgio F. Coloni, MD[a]

KEYWORDS

- Emphysema • COPD • Lung volume reduction
- Respiratory failure • Bridge to transplantation
- Residual volume

Emphysema is characterized by a permanent and irreversible enlargement of air spaces distal to the terminal bronchiole accompanied by destruction of their walls without fibrosis.[1] Notwithstanding the improvements in understanding the pathophysiology of the disease and the effectiveness of medical therapy, it continues to be a major source of morbidity and mortality in developed countries. Despite all the available therapies, the course of the disease is progressively disabling with a significant increase in overall morbidity and mortality. Over the past 50 years many investigators have attempted to determine which factors influence survival of patients who have chronic obstructive pulmonary disease (COPD). When the forced expiratory volume in 1 second (FEV_1) is less than 30% of the predicted value, less than 50% of patients will survive for 3 years[2,3] despite optimal medical therapy; thus, medical treatment certainly shows some limitations in the most advanced phases of the disease.

Various surgical procedures have been proposed in the past to relieve dyspnea and improve quality of life in patients who have advanced emphysema; however, bullectomy is the only operation that has stood the test of time. Lung transplantation and lung volume reduction surgery (LVRS) are now established treatment modalities in selected patients.

Despite controversies, LVRS has been shown to be beneficial to selected patients who have end-stage emphysema.[4,5] This operation was rescued by Cooper and associates[6] in the early 1990s and progressively gained acceptance. The basic principle of this procedure is that removal of the most diseased parts of the hyperinflated lungs contributes to remodeling and restoring the chest wall and diaphragmatic mechanics during breathing. There is no doubt that LVRS allows a significant functional improvement in a selected group of patients; however, it still carries a substantial morbidity, even if mortality is low at the centers with more experience.[7] Patients who have the most advanced functional deterioration show a higher surgical mortality and less impressive functional results, suggesting that LVRS should be considered more carefully in these situations.[8] In particular, patients who have very low FEV_1 and either homogeneous emphysema or a very low DLCO are at high risk for death, and the most recently published data have indicated that patients who have non–upper lobe disease have a higher operative mortality.

[a] Università di Roma "La Sapienza," Cattedra di Chirurgia Toracica, Policlinico Umberto I, V.le del Policlinico 166, 00100 Rome, Italy
[b] Universita di Roma "La Sapienza," Cattedra di Chirurgia Toracica, Ospedale S. Andrea, V.le del Policlinico 166, 00100 Rome, Italy
* Corresponding author.
E-mail address: federico.venuta@uniroma1.it (F. Venuta).

Thorac Surg Clin 19 (2009) 255–260
doi:10.1016/j.thorsurg.2009.04.002

Bronchoscopic alternatives to the surgical approach have been recently proposed and some of them could play an important role in the future; in particular, bronchoscopic lung volume reduction with one-way valves is on the way to clinical application.

Several procedures have been described experimentally and in selected clinical settings with the use of occlusive stents, synthetic sealants, and unidirectional valves.[9–13] These procedures were all designed to reduce hyperinflation and obtain atelectasis of the most destroyed functionless parts of the emphysematous lungs (heterogeneous emphysema). They have been evaluated to find safe alternatives to LVRS, especially for patients who have the most advanced disease.

It has been postulated that blocking an airway supplying the most overinflated emphysematous parts of the lung could induce partial or complete atelectasis of these regions mimicking LVRS and contributing to alleviating symptoms. This result was experimentally demonstrated by Ingenito and colleagues[13] in 2001; this experimental work clearly demonstrates the functional effectiveness of bronchoscopic exclusion of lung segments. Ingenito studied three groups of sheep with papain-induced emphysema and compared the effectiveness of surgical lung volume reduction, bronchoscopic lung volume reduction performed by occluding lung segments with a synthetic sealant, and a sham procedure that was a simple bronchoscopy. The results of this experimental work showed that bronchial occlusion can produce the same functional results as LVRS.

Instead of sealants, other authors have used endobronchial devices working as one-way valves. These devices allow air to exit from the lung parenchyma but not to enter and should also allow a sufficient clearance of bronchial secretions.

There are basically two devices under clinical evaluation: the Spiration umbrella and the Emphasys one-way valve. These devices are placed in the segmental or subsegmental bronchi to obtain lobar exclusion. The goal of the procedure is deflation of the target area in patients who have heterogeneous emphysema, mimicking surgical lung volume reduction.

Collateral ventilation plays an important role in the success of these procedures. Collateral ventilation is defined as the ability of gas to move from one part of the lung to another through nonanatomic pathways. It was first described by Van Allen and colleagues[14] in 1930; they obstructed sublobar bronchi in canine lungs and noted no collapse distal to the obstruction. They used the term "collateral respiration" to explain how gases may enter one lobule from another in the lung without resorting to known anatomic pathways. Hogg and colleagues[15] demonstrated that resistance to collateral airflow in postmortem emphysematous human lungs was low compared with normal lungs, concluding that collateral channels may be important ventilatory pathways in emphysema. Terry and coworkers[16] studied collateral ventilation in normal subjects and subjects who had emphysema. In young normal people they found that resistance to collateral ventilation is high at functional residual capacity and they concluded that in these subjects there was a negligible role for collateral channels in the distribution of ventilation. Patients who had emphysema had lower resistance through collateral channels than through the airways. Already at that time it was postulated that those results may have startling therapeutic implications.[17] Collateral ventilation is present in normal lungs but it does not play an important role; in emphysematous lungs the destruction of alveolar septa creates a preferential route for collateral air flow. Gunnarson and coworkers[18] looked in detail at patients who had COPD undergoing general anesthesia; they described significantly less atelectasis and shunt when compared with the population with normal lungs. Three levels of collateral ventilation have been described in human lungs from the anatomic point of view. Kohn first described intra-alveolar pores more than a century ago; in 1955, Lambert[19] described accessory bronchiolar-alveolar connections; interbronchial channels were described by Martin in dogs, and have been subsequently verified in humans.[20] Morrell and colleagues[21] discovered that segmental collateral ventilation occurred to a much greater extent in the emphysematous lung than in the normal lung. Although surprisingly not described in the most recent reviews,[20,22] the older medical literature provides some support for the concept of poorly characterized interlobar communications.[23] Using careful dissection techniques and selective lobar intubation, Hogg and colleagues[15] noted complete upper/lower lobe fissures in only 3 of 8 normal lungs and 1 of 8 emphysematous lungs, with substantial flow across the incomplete fissures. Rosenberg and Lyons[24] examined 13 isolated lungs from patients who had various diseases, including one patient who had emphysema and pneumonia with significant cross-lobar flow. Their microscopic analysis of the regions adjacent to the fissures where interlobar collateral flow had been seen demonstrated lobar/alveolar pores, potentially variants of the pores of Kohn. Such interlobar flow and communications were not observed in pediatric lungs. It has been speculated that pathologic collaterals may represent inflammatory or sheer force damage between airways and the parenchyma and serve to even out areas on inhomogeneity.[20,22]

The presence of a generous collateral ventilation at an intra- and extralobar level reduces the effectiveness of lobar exclusion with one-way valves; refilling of the obstructed segments prevents atelectasis and volume reduction. Prediction of existence of complete interlobar fissures is thus crucial to improve results.

The first-generation Emphasys endobronchial valve (EBV) (Emphasys, Redwood City, California) is an endobronchial device designed to control and redirect airflow (**Fig. 1**). It is a one-way, polymer, duckbill valve mounted inside a stainless steel cylinder attached to a nickel-titanium (nitinol) self-expanding retainer. It prevents air from entering the target lung but allows air and mucus to exit. The first generation of valves was provided in three sizes, each intended for a different range of target bronchial lumen diameters: 4.0 to 5.5 mm (inner–outer diameter), 5.0 to 7.0 mm, and 6.5 to 8.5 mm; the valve is 10 mm long. These valves are placed in the operating room, with the patient intubated under intravenous anesthesia (propofol infusion) and spontaneous assisted ventilation. After the patient is intubated, the flexible bronchoscope is advanced into the endotracheal tube and the target bronchi (usually segmental or subsegmental) are chosen. They correspond to the most hyperinflated part of the lung affected by heterogeneous emphysema, as evaluated by CT and V/Q scans. A guide wire is inserted through the operating channel of the bronchoscope and left in place while the bronchoscope is withdrawn; a flexible delivery catheter is guided to the target bronchus by the guide wire. Local anesthesia is generously administered before inserting the valves to prevent coughing. The fiberoptic bronchoscope is reinserted after the advancement of the delivery catheter; the tip of the delivery catheter containing the valve is pushed with a gentle rotation in the selected bronchial orifice, and the valve is delivered. Fiberoptic bronchoscopy performed after removal of the delivery catheter confirms the correct placement of the valve. Gentle suction through the bronchoscope ensures the correct opening of the valve to allow deflation of the lung and clearance of secretions. No fluoroscopy is required. The valves can be removed easily if placement is not satisfactory using a rat-tooth grasper through the working channel of the bronchoscope. The EBV can be clearly seen at chest radiograph.

The first generation of EBVs have been extensively used in several prospective, nonrandomized, single center longitudinal pilot studies to evaluate safety and short-term efficacy with promising results in a selected group of patients who had heterogeneous end-stage emphysema.

A new generation of EBVs is ready and is currently under evaluation in a multicenter prospective trial: the Zephyr endobronchial valve (**Fig. 2**). This new valve is a device incorporating a one-way valve supported by a stent-like self-expanding retainer that secures the EBV in place during all physiologic conditions, including coughing. The retainer is a self-expanding tubular mesh

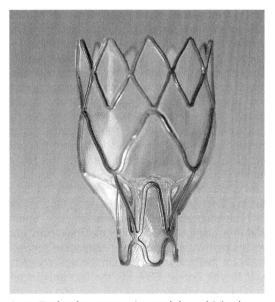

Fig. 2. Zephyr last-generation endobronchial valve.

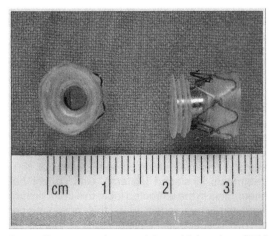

Fig. 1. First-generation endobronchial valve (EBV) designed to control and redirect air flow.

structure that is cut from nitinol superelastic alloy tubing and processed to its final expanded dimensions. It is covered with silicone to create a seal between the implant and the bronchial wall; the silicone membrane is formed integrally with the struts of the self-expanding retainer component. When the EBV is delivered into the target bronchus, the retainer expands to contact the walls of the lumen. Also this valve has been designed to allow air to be vented from the isolated lung segment while preventing air from refilling the isolated lung area during inspiration; it vents during expiration and closes when flow is reversed during inhalation. The Zephyr EBV is provided in two sizes: the EBV 4.0 designed for bronchial lumens with diameters of 4.0 mm to 7.0 mm, and the Zephyr EBV 5.5 designed for bronchial lumens with diameters of 5.5 mm to 8.5 mm. The previous version of the device was provided in three different sizes for the same overall treatable lumen diameter range of 4.0 to 8.5 mm. The larger diameter of the new-generation valve can sometimes be suitable to lobar bronchi.

The performance of the valve is different according to the type of valve (first generation versus second generation of EBV), and to the size of the device itself. The cracking pressure, and thus flow resistance, was higher for the EBV of the first generation when compared with the Zephyr valve. Within the two different models of valves, flow resistance is lower for valves of the larger diameter. Air expiratory flow is much higher for large valves of the second generation.

A flexible delivery catheter is also used to place this second-generation EBV to the targeted bronchial lumen. The catheter is constructed of a flexible stainless steel and polymer composite shaft. It has an actuation handle on the proximal end and a retractable polymer housing for containing the compressed Zephyr EBV on the distal end. A bronchial diameter measurement gauge made of flexible polymer is attached to the proximal end of the distal housing. This measurement gauge allows the user to visually (bronchoscopically) measure the diameter of the bronchial lumen before device deployment to verify that the size gauge of the valve is appropriate for the target lumen. The measurement gauge consists of two sets of flexible gauges. On the delivery catheter for the Zephyr EBV 4.0 the larger gauge spans a 7-mm diameter and the smaller gage spans a 4-mm diameter, indicating the maximum and minimum treatable bronchial diameters respectively for this size of device. On the delivery catheter for the Zephyr EBV 5.5, the two gauges are sized to span diameters of 8.5 mm and 5.5 mm. The EBV is compressed into the retractable distal

housing by the operator using a specifically designed EBV loader system. The loaded catheter is advanced to the target location and the valve is deployed by actuating the deployment handle, which retracts the distal housing and releases the EBV. The delivery catheter is designed to be inserted through a 2.8-mm diameter working channel of a flexible bronchoscope. This new generation of valves can thus be placed under local anesthesia because the deployment maneuver is much simpler.

After a series of animal experiments, more than 100 patients have been treated so far in pilot studies performed at several centers worldwide, with selection criteria similar to those for LVRS. All patients had heterogeneous emphysema with clear target areas. The first 10 patients treated with a first-generation type of EBV were reported by Snell and colleagues.[25] They demonstrated that that type of bronchoscopic prosthesis could be safely and reliably placed into the human bronchi; however, symptomatic improvement was observed only in 4 patients, with no major change in radiographic findings, lung function, or 6-minute walk distance at 1 month, although base transfer improved from 7.47 ± 2.0 to 8.26 ± 2.6 mL/min/mm Hg and nuclear upper lobe perfusion fell from $32\% \pm 10\%$ to $27\% \pm 9\%$. Toma and colleagues[26] subsequently reported on 8 patients undergoing unilateral volume reduction with a second generation of EBV. Five patients had emphysema judged too severe for volume reduction surgery and 3 refused the operation. After valve placement there was a 34% increase in FEV_1 and 29% difference in DLCO; CT scans showed a substantial reduction in regional volume in 4 of the 8 patients. The same group also reported that in a subgroup of patients in whom invasive measurements were performed, improvement in exercise capacity was associated with a reduction of lung compliance and isotime esophageal pressure-time product.[27] Two other series of patients treated with EBV have been reported.[28,29] Overall, all patients tolerated the treatment well. Between three and five valves were placed in the target lobe and most of them received unilateral treatment. It has been demonstrated that the procedure can be safely performed with encouraging short-term results.

In our experience[29] we observed one contralateral and two bilateral pneumothoraxes out of 17 treatments (2 staged bilateral). One patient had pneumonia in the untreated lobe; this complication was easily managed with the administration of broad-spectrum antibiotics. The functional improvement was statistically significant; in particular FEV_1 markedly improved and the residual volume decreased. At 3 months more than 50% of the patients still show at least a 30% functional improvement; most of them required less supplemental oxygen and 7 out of 15 were able to stop it. We were not able to observe a complete atelectasis of the lobe where valves were implanted, although this has been described by other authors. In most of the patients, the shape of the chest was redesigned. Exercise tolerance was also improved and remained stable after 3 months of follow-up. Contralateral bronchoscopic lung volume reduction (BLVR) could be attempted to obtain a second functional improvement when pulmonary function tests start to deteriorate again, as it is done for LVRS. A contralateral BLVR was performed in 2 of our patients, but neither was required for functional reasons. Both patients had pneumothorax on the contralateral side and valves were placed with the aim of stopping the air leak; this result was easily obtained, along with further functional improvement. With more experience, simultaneous bilateral insertion of the valves could be attempted. One of the advantages of the endobronchial lung volume reduction is that the procedure can be reversed and other treatments tried if necessary.

A cumulative review of the first 98 cases[30] performed at different institutions has been recently published. This report focused on an extremely heterogeneous group of patients; however, it clearly showed that a greater magnitude of improvement could be obtained in patients with lobar exclusion and unilateral lobar placement. Patients with baseline FEV_1 less than 30% and residual volume greater than 225% of predicted showed a significant functional improvement. Overall, 46% of the patients had clinically significant improvement in FEV_1 (greater than 15%) and 55% had improvement of greater than 15% or 50 m for the 6-minute walking test 90 days after the procedure. In that study various patient subgroups were treated with different treatment strategies; this aspect should be standardized in any upcoming prospective trial.

The short-term results with BLVR are encouraging, but long-term follow-up is required, as well as multicenter trials, to evaluate the therapeutic potential of this procedure.

REFERENCES

1. Russi EW, De Wever W, Decramer M. Surgery for emphysema: medical aspects. In: Verleden GM, Van Raemdonck D, Leryt T, et al, editors. Surgery for non neoplastic disorders of the chest: a clinical update. European Respiratory Society Monograph 2004;29(9):129–38.

2. Anthonisen NR, Wright EC, Hodgkin JE, IPPB Trial Group. Prognosis in chronic obstructive pulmonary disease. Am Rev Respir Dis 1986;133:14–20.

3. Ries AL, Kaplan RM, Limberg TM, et al. Effects of pulmonary rehabilitation on physiologic and psychosocial outcomes in patients with chronic obstructive pulmonary disease. Ann Intern Med 1995;122:823–32.

4. Yusen RD, Lefrak SS, Gierada DS, et al. A prospective evaluation of lung volume reduction surgery in 200 consecutive patients. Chest 2003;123:1026–37.

5. Ciccone AM, Meyers BF, Guthrie TJ, et al. Long term outcome of bilateral lung volume reduction in 250 consecutive patients with emphysema. J Thorac Cardiovasc Surg 2003;125:513–25.

6. Cooper JD, Trulock EP, Triantafillou AN, et al. Bilateral pneumectomy (volume reduction) for chronic obstructive pulmonary disease. J Thorac Cardiovasc Surg 1995;109:106–19.

7. Fishman A, Martinez F, Naunheim K, et al. National Emphysema Treatment Trial Research Group. A randomized trial comparing lung volume reduction surgery with medical therapy for emphysema. N Engl J Med 2003;348:2059–73.

8. National Emphysema Treatment Trial Research Group. Patients at high risk of death after lung volume reduction surgery. N Engl J Med 2001;345:1075–83.

9. Lausberg HF, Chino K, Patterson GA, et al. Bronchial fenestration improves expiratory flow in emphysematous human lungs. Ann Thorac Surg 2003;75:393–8.

10. Snell GI, Smith GA, Silovers AJ, et al. Bronchoscopic volume reduction: a pilot study [paper 25]. ACCP Meeting. Tampa (FL), March 21–24, 2001.

11. Sabanhatan S, Richardson J, Pieri – Davies S. Bronchoscopic lung volume reduction. J Cardiovasc Surg 2003;44:101–8.

12. Fann JI, Berry GJ, Burden TA. Bronchoscopic approach to lung volume reduction using a valve device. J Bronchol 2003;10:253–9.

13. Ingenito EP, Reilly JJ, Mentzer SJ, et al. Bronchoscopic volume reduction: a safe and effective alternative to surgical therapy for emphysema. Am J Respir Crit Care Med 2001;164:295–301.

14. Van Allen CM, Lindskog GE, Richter HT. Gaseous interchange between adjacent lung lobules. Yale J Biol Med 1930;2:297–300.

15. Hogg JC, Macklem PT, Thurlbeck WM. The resistance of collateral channels in excised human lungs. J Clin Invest 1969;48:421–31.

16. Terry PB, Traystman RJ, Newball HH, et al. Collateral ventilation in man. N Engl J Med 1978;298:10–5.

17. Macklem PT. Collateral ventilation. N Engl J Med 1978;298:49–50.

18. Gunnarsson L, Tokics L, Lundquist H, et al. Chronic obstructive pulmonary disease and anaesthesia: formation of atelectasis and gas exchange impairment. Eur Respir J 1991;4:1106–16.

19. Lambert MW. Accessory bronchoalveolar communications. J Pathol Bacteriol 1955;70:311–4.
20. Mitzner W. Collateral ventilation. In: Crystal RG, editor. The lung: scientific foundations. New York: Raven press; 1991. p. 1053–63.
21. Morrell NW, Wignall BK, Biggs T, et al. Collateral ventilation and gas exchange in emphysema. Am J Respir Crit Care Med 1994;150:635–41.
22. Delaunois L. Anatomy and physiology of collateral ventilation in man. Eur Respir J 1989;2:893–904.
23. Fraser RG, Peter JA, Pare PD, et al. Diagnosis of diseases of the chest. Philadelphia: WB Saunders Company; 1988. p. 476–8.
24. Rosenberg DF, Lyons HA. Collateral ventilation in excised human lungs. Respiration 1979;37:125–34.
25. Snell GI, Halsworth L, Borrill ZL, et al. The potential for bronchoscopic lung volume reduction using bronchial prosthesis: a pilot study. Chest 2003;124: 1073–80.
26. Toma TP, Hopkinson NS, Hiller J, et al. Bronchoscopic volume reduction with valve implants in patients with severe emphysema. Lancet 2003; 361:931–3.
27. Hopkinsons NS, Toma TP, Hansell DM, et al. Effect of bronchoscopic lung volume reduction on dynamic hyperinflation and exercise in emphysema. Am J Respir Crit Care Med 2005;171:423–4.
28. Yim AP, Hwong TM, Lee TW, et al. Early results of endoscopic lung volume reduction for emphysema. J Thorac Cardiovasc Surg 2004;127:1564–73.
29. Venuta F, De Giacomo T, Rendina EA, et al. Bronchoscopic lung volume reduction with one way valves in patients with emphysema. Ann Thorac Surg 2005; 79:411–7.
30. Yim IYP, Toma T, Geddes DM, et al. Bronchoscopic lung volume reduction for end stage emphysema; report on the first 98 patients. Chest 2006;129: 518–26.

Update on Donor Assessment, Resuscitation, and Acceptance Criteria, Including Novel Techniques— Non–Heart-Beating Donor Lung Retrieval and Ex Vivo Donor Lung Perfusion

Jonathan C. Yeung, MD[a], Marcelo Cypel, MD[a],
Thomas K. Waddell, MD[a], Dirk van Raemdonck, MD[b],
Shaf Keshavjee, MD[a],*

KEYWORDS

- Lung transplantation • Non-heart beating donor
- Ex vivo lung perfusion • Donor assessment
- Donor resuscitation

Lung transplantation has seen increasing success as a therapy that improves the quality and quantity of life for selected patients who have end-stage lung disease.[1] Only a minority of patients, however, can benefit because of the lack of acceptable donor organs.

The largest source of donor organs is from donations after neurologic determination of death (DNDDs). Unfortunately, because of injuries acquired during the process of brain death, the average organ procurement rate remains disappointing. United Network for Organ Sharing data reveal that only 2489 individual lungs were transplanted from 8089 deceased donors in 2007.[2] As a comparison, 11,752 individual kidneys were transplanted from that same pool of organ donors.

This lack of donor organs has been the impetus for the search for alternative donor sources. A common strategy to maximize use of DNDD lungs has been to transplant extended criteria donor organs (ie, those organs that fall outside of International Society for Heart and Lung Transplantation [ISHLT] standard criteria but still believed to be transplantable).[3] Some transplant programs have begun to explore the use of circulation-arrested

[a] Toronto Lung Transplant Program, Toronto General Hospital, 200 Elizabeth Street, Toronto, ON, Canada
[b] The Lung Transplant Program, University Hospital Gasthuisberg, UZ Gasthuisberg, Herestraat 49, Leuven 3000, Belgium
* Corresponding author. Division of Thoracic Surgery, Toronto General Hospital, 200 Elizabeth Street, 9N-947, Toronto, ON, Canada.
E-mail address: shaf.keshavjee@uhn.on.ca (S. Keshavjee).

Thorac Surg Clin 19 (2009) 261–274
doi:10.1016/j.thorsurg.2009.02.006

donors, so called non–heart-beating donors (NHBDs) or donors after cardiac death,[4,5] as alternative sources for lungs. Because most patients succumb as a result of cardiac arrest, the use of NHBDs could open a new pool of donor organs of such magnitude that ultimately the entire demand could be met.

A major problem with the use of extended criteria donor organs and NHBDs is the difficulty in assessing which lungs can be used safely. The urgency during the retrieval of lungs from NHBDs compounds this difficulty.[6] This article focuses on DNDD and NHBD lung criteria, assessment, preservation, retrieval, and the possible role of ex vivo lung perfusion (EVLP).

INTERNATIONAL SOCIETY FOR HEART AND LUNG TRANSPLANTATION ACCEPTANCE CRITERIA

One major reason for the poor organ procurement rate is the difficulty of accurately judging lungs as safe for transplantation during donor evaluation. The ISHLT criteria (**Box 1**) utlining ideal donors are strict and generally based on clinical impressions formed during the development of lung transplantation rather than on medical evidence.[7] These criteria are assessed during organ retrieval and are based on donor history, arterial blood gases, chest radiography, bronchoscopy, and physical examination of the lung. This clinical

---

> **Box 1**
> **Standard International Society for Heart and Lung Transplantation donor lung criteria**
>
> Age <55 years
>
> Clear serial chest radiograph
>
> Normal gas exchange ($Pao_2 > 300$ mm Hg on $Fio_2 = 1.0$, positive end-expiratory pressure [PEEP] 5 cm H_2O)
>
> Absence of chest trauma
>
> No evidence of aspiration or sepsis
>
> Absence of purulent secretions at bronchoscopy
>
> Absence of organisms on sputum Gram's stain
>
> No history of primary pulmonary disease or active pulmonary infection
>
> Tobacco history <20 pack years
>
> ABO blood-group compatibility
>
> Appropriate size match with prospective recipient
>
> *Data from* Orens JB, Boehler A, de Perrot M, et al. A review of lung transplant donor acceptability criteria. J Heart Lung Transplant 2003;22(11):1183–200.

---

evaluation is imprecise and approximately 11% to 57% of lungs go on to primary graft dysfunction (PGD) of varying severity, some of which may be the result of unrecognized donor injury.[8] As a consequence, transplant clinicians remain conservative when choosing lungs for fear of potential PGD. It is estimated that 40% of rejected donor lungs could be used safely if more detailed and accurate evaluation were available to identify these lungs.[9]

NON–HEART-BEATING DONORS

At the First International Workshop on NHBD, held in Maastricht, the Netherlands, in 1995, four types of donors were identified, the so-called Maastricht categories.[10] Categories I (dead on arrival) and II (unsuccessful resuscitation) comprise the uncontrolled donors. Categories III (awaiting cardiac arrest) and IV (cardiac arrest in brain-dead donors) include the controlled donors (see **Box 1**).

The first clinical lung transplantation, performed by James Hardy in 1963,[11] used a lung from a NHBD who died from a myocardial infarction. At that time, use of a NHBD was a necessity, as the concept of brain death was not yet legally established. Once brain death had reached the status of general acceptance in the 1970s,[12] all organs were harvested from brain-dead donors who had intact circulation.

Renewed interest in the potential use of lungs from NHBDs followed a series of experiments in dogs by Egan and coworkers in the early 1990s.[13,14] This group demonstrated that lung cells remain viable for a certain period after circulatory arrest.[15,16] The lung is the sole solid organ that is not dependent on perfusion for aerobic metabolism but instead uses a mechanism of passive diffusion through the alveoli for substrate delivery. Many experimental studies continued to investigate the possibility of using lungs from NHBDs for transplantation.[17,18]

Clinically, the first explicit description of the use of lungs from a NHBD derives from Love and colleagues[19] in 1995 (n = 3). This series, using lungs from category III donors, was updated in 2003 (n = 20).[20] In 2001, Steen reported successful lung transplantation using a category II NHBD who died in hospital after failed resuscitation after myocardial infarction.[6] In 2004, the group from Andres Varela[21] in Madrid reported two successful lung transplantations from out-of-hospital NHBDs (category I). This series has been updated (n = 17).[22,23] Several centers worldwide have adopted NHBD programs in their clinical routine of lung transplantation. All reported series deal with controlled donation after withdrawal from life support (category III).[24–27] The total experience in this category amounts to nearly 100 patients worldwide.

LUNG ASSESSMENT

After declaration of brain death, consent for donation is discussed with relatives and, when available, donor registries can be checked. Blood samples are obtained to check the blood group and to minimize the risk for donor-transmitted diseases. A chest radiograph is taken to exclude gross parenchymal or pleural abnormalities. A CT scan of the lungs may be available from patients who spent time in a critical care unit. A bronchoscopy should be performed to exclude gross infection or anatomic abnormalities. Finally, gas exchange capacity of the donor lungs can be assessed with an oxygen challenge. A retrieval surgeon performs a direct evaluation by macroscopic observation and palpation to assess lung compliance and edema. Palpation also is used to exclude intrinsic lung disease, areas of contusion, pneumonic infiltrates, or nodules before finally accepting the lungs. Observation of the ventilated lungs during deflation is important to assess acceptable elastic recoil, especially if donors have a smoking history.

Donor lung assessment in controlled (category III) NHBDs can be done in the hours before planned termination of life support identical to the situation in DNDD donors. The situation in uncontrolled donors, however, is different as no previous medical history and no serologic, radiographic, bronchoscopic, or functional data are available at the time of circulatory arrest. This information, legal permission, and family consent are to be obtained in the hours thereafter. In the meantime, the lungs can be topically cooled for several hours by inserting chest drains for infusion of a cold preservation solution.[28,29] Viability testing of a potentially damaged graft is mandatory so that only NHBD lungs of good quality are transplanted. Gas exchange capacity can be assessed in situ with lungs ventilated using a pulmonary artery flush with 300 mL of heparinized venous blood drained from the donor while they are on arteriovenous extracorporeal membrane oxygenation (ECMO)[23] or by using an ex vivo ventilation and reperfusion circuit (described later).[6,30]

NON–HEART-BEATING DONORS LUNG RETRIEVAL

In contrast to brain-dead donors, a warm ischemic period is added to the cold ischemic interval. An untouched donor lung can tolerate a warm ischemic period for up to 60 min in the cadaver.[31] This time interval is sufficient to insert drains for topical cooling in uncontrolled donors and for opening the sternum and pericardium for flush cooling in controlled donors.

In category IV donors, in whom the heart stops prematurely during organ retrieval (in brain-dead patients) before aortic cross clamp and cardioplegia, a cannula can be inserted rapidly in the pulmonary artery for cold flush perfusion.

In category III donors, life support is withdrawn by switching off the ventilator (or extubation), and spontaneous cardiac arrest can be awaited in the operating room or in the ICU with immediate transport of the donor to the operating room after certification of death. The use of heparin before circulatory arrest is practiced by some teams although this does not seem a problem if not allowed.[25] A hands-off period of 3 to 5 minutes is required in most NHBD protocols to assure that no spontaneous recovery of heart activity takes place. The donor then is certified dead by one (or more) physicians not involved in the transplant team. Practices vary widely between countries because of variations in local legal requirements and ethical approval.[32]

In category I and category II donors, after failed resuscitation and certification of death, chest tubes are inserted for topical lung cooling[6,23] and patients can be connected to an arteriovenous ECMO system via catheters inserted in the groin for preservation of abdominal organs.[23]

After reintubation of the donor and sternotomy, both lungs are quickly inspected. The pericardium is opened and the main pulmonary artery is incised and its lumen inspected for gross thrombi that can be extracted. A cannula then is inserted and secured, followed by an anterograde flush with 60 mL/kg of cold Perfadex (Vitrolife, Gothenburg, Sweden) with the lungs ventilated. The heart then is extracted and an additional retrograde flush is delivered via the four pulmonary veins with 1 L of the same solution to evacuate possible microthrombi. The lungs then are excised, carefully inspected, packed in three sterile bags and transported in the usual manner. The transplantation to be performed is not different from that using lungs recovered from heart-beating donors. The total ischemic time starts from the moment of circulatory arrest in the donor (or systemic blood pressure <40 mm Hg) until the time of reperfusion of the lungs.

NON–HEART-BEATING DONORS CRITERIA

The criteria for accepting a lung from a NHBD does not differ from the standard criteria (**Box 2**) used for lungs from brain-dead donors.[7,33] The ultimate judgment as to whether or not a donor lung is used for transplantation is made on the basis of donor and recipient factors in individual cases. In a NHBD, the mode of cardiac death[34] and the length of the agonal period[35] before the circulation ceases may negatively influence the quality of the organ before any preservation methods can be initiated. These factors also should be taken into account when evaluating a NHBD lung.

Not all patients who have an irrecoverable neurologic outcome and who are admitted to a critical care unit when a decision is made to stop life support qualify for potential NHBD category III, as some have been hospitalized and ventilated for many days and may suffer from infection, especially pneumonia.

EXTENSION OF DONOR CRITERIA

Although the best transplant outcomes occur when ideal organs are matched carefully to ideal recipients, the shortage of donor organs causes a high waitlist morbidity and mortality. To maximize the use of DNDD donors, many centers, in particular those with more experience, have been using donors outside the standard ISHLT criteria.[36] Common liberalization of donor criteria includes using lungs from donors aged greater than 55, who have smoking history of more than 20 pack years, who have been on a ventilator more than 4 days, or who have positive Gram's stain on bronchoalveolar lavage. Absolute contraindications to organ donation remain situations that carry a risk for disease transmission from donor to recipient, such as sepsis, active extra-central nervous system malignancy, and positive serology for HIV.

A series of articles examining the use of "marginal" or "extended criteria" donor lungs have been published showing mostly equivalent short-term outcomes.[37–43] Each group used different criteria, however, to define an extended criteria donor organ, making comparison difficult.

These characteristics are summarized in **Table 1**. Bronchoscopic and chest radiograph evaluation remain the most subjective of the ISHLT criteria and it is within these criteria that there is evidence of an increased risk for postoperative death. In 2002, Pierre and colleagues[42] reported on experience with 63 extended criteria donor organs for which part of the extended criteria included chest radiographic infiltrates and purulent secretions on bronchoscopy. Within this series, there was a statistically significantly higher 30- and 90-day mortality when compared with recipients of standard criteria donor organs during the same timeframe. Of the six recipient deaths believed related to the quality of the donor lung, three had purulent secretions at bronchoscopy and five had chest x-ray (CXR) infiltrates. This experience demonstrated that donor lungs with truly purulent secretions and bilateral infiltrates clearly are at higher risk and should not be used. A series by Lardinois and colleagues in 2005 showed equivalent 30-day and 1-year survival rates in recipients of ideal lungs and recipients of marginal lungs.[41] A subgroup analysis, however, suggested that recipients of lungs with purulent secretions and a Pao_2 less than 300 had a negative impact on outcome. Gabbay and colleagues[39] reported on a series in which 39 lungs with abnormal CXR and 24 lungs with infection were used. Although they showed equivalent 30-day survival rates in marginal donors and ideal donors after transplant, infection was defined as purulent secretions or positive Gram's stain; the amount of purulent secretions on bronchoscopy was not reported. They did not transplant lungs with evidence of severe pulmonary infection. Thus, judgment of the severity of abnormal CXR or bronchoscopy remains important in ensuring good outcomes.

Other factors also should be considered when extended criteria donor lungs are used. In the Gabbay series, graft ischemic times were predictive of recipient Pao_2/Fio_2 (P/F) ratio.[39] The investigators did not transplant marginal lungs that had ischemic times greater than 6 hours. The Pierre series showed that recipients of advanced age or who had *Burkholderia cepacia* colonization had higher organ-specific mortality with the use of extended criteria donor lungs.[42] Sundaresan and colleagues[43] reported a higher need to use cardiopulmonary bypass to facilitate implantation of the second graft when using extended criteria donor lungs, indicating that there is some lung dysfunction inherent in the use of such lungs. Thus, the investigators have suggested that single lung transplants using marginal lungs should occur in

Table 1
Summary of extended donor criteria and survival rates

First Author and Reference No.	No. of Transplants	Extended Criteria Donor Organs Used	30-Day Survival (Ext/Ideal)	1-Year Survival (Ext/Ideal)	Age >55	Smoking >20 y	Abnormal Chest X-Ray	Pao$_2$ <300	Positive Gram's Stain	Pus/Aspiration	Ventilation >5d
Bhorade[37]	113	52 (46%)	88%/80%[a]	84%/72%	9	15	5	0	0	0	7
Gabbay[39]	140	64 (57%)	96%/92%	87%/78%	4	5	39	20[b]	24	0	NR
Sundaresan[43]	133	44 (33%)	100%/96.6%	NR	2	9	34	6	NR	0	NR
Kron[40]	26	10 (35%)	90%/NR	NR	NR	NR	6	0	NR	4	0
Pierre[42]	128	63 (51%)	82.5%/93.8%	NR	9	26	41	0	NR	8	NR
Botha[38]	201	83 (41%)	84.3%/91.5%	NR	17	32	21	11	NR	14	19
Aigner[33]	94	23 (24%)	92.3%/88.9%	84.6%/81.9%	5	1	3	8	NR	0	NR
Lardinois[41]	148	63 (43%)	93.7%/90.6%	81%/83.5%	12	20	29	15	NR	14	NR

Abbreviations: Ext, extended; NR, not reported.
[a] Hospital survival (approximately 13 days).
[b] Pao$_2$ > 300 after donor management.

emphysema, when the native lung can continue to contribute to oxygenation, versus in fibrotic lung disease, when the native lung may not.

Overall, many of the criteria for ideal donors do not seem to affect outcome in multiple series from different centers. For centers with long waiting lists and limited donor pools, there is a role for thoughtful use of donor lungs that do not fit the ISHLT donor criteria.

DONOR LUNG EVALUATION SCORING

The acceptance criteria for donor lungs are largely clinical and the decision to use a donor lung, especially an extended criteria donor lung, hinges on the experience of the retrieval surgeon. These criteria thus are largely subjective and suffer from high interobserver variability. To better standardize donor lung assessment across lung transplant programs, a donor lung score was introduced by Oto and colleagues.[44] This score has five domains representing the major clinical criteria for donor lung assessment: age, smoking history, CXR, secretions, and P/F ratio. P/F ratio was prospectively given a double weighting because of its clinical significance. Using a prospectively collected initial cohort of 87 donors in 2001 and a retrospectively collected lung transplant validation cohort of 157 patients from 2002 to 2005, it was found that medically unsuitable lungs resulted in a higher donor score and that early post-transplant outcomes were significantly associated with higher donor scores. This group is planning a larger prospective study to further validate the scoring system. Cypel and colleagues,[45] however, recently applied the donor score retrospectively to the Toronto Lung Transplant Program in a larger number of patients and failed to find a similar correlation between donor score and early post-transplant outcomes. Despite this result, refining this lung scoring system to be effective prospectively and across programs would be invaluable for predicting lung outcome, comparing donor lung quality worldwide, and maintaining comparable research databases.

MOLECULAR EVALUATION

Clinical evaluation, informally or with a specific donor scoring system, remains dependent on clinical criteria that are not evidence based and are subject to significant interobserver variability. With improvements in the understanding of donor lung biology and concomitant advances in technology, novel markers of donor lung assessment are being investigated for clinical use. High levels of inflammatory mediators at the time of

reperfusion can predispose the lung to ischemia-reperfusion injury, a major contributor of PGD.[46] There is a high potential for activation of inflammatory parameters during the process of brain death and organ retrieval. Many of these patients sustain major trauma, intracranial bleeding, and sustained mechanical ventilation, which all have been shown to lead to increased systemic inflammation and lung injury.[47,48] In addition, brain death itself induces an inflammatory reaction and cytokine storm.[49] As such, markers of inflammation recently have been investigated to assess organ suitability for transplantation. de Perrot and colleagues[50] showed that interleukin (IL)-8 levels in donor lung tissue before and after transplantation increased with time after reperfusion and that patients who have severe PGD had significantly higher IL-8 levels during ischemia and after reperfusion. Fisher and colleagues[51] studied the levels of IL-8 in BAL fluid from 26 donor lungs used for transplantation and showed that a high concentration of IL-8 in donor bronchoalveolar lavage fluid was correlated with severe graft dysfunction and with early postoperative deaths. To further study the predictive value of proinflammatory cytokines, Kaneda and colleagues[52] used real-time polymerase chain reaction (RT-PCR) to study the levels of IL-6, IL-1β, IL-8, IL-10, interferon-γ, and tumor necrosis factor (TNF)-α in donor lung biopsies at end of cold ischemia. They found that the IL-6/IL-10 ratio in the donor lung before the time of implantation was predictive of recipient 30-day mortality. Thus, rapid RT-PCR could be used as a tool to predict donor lung outcomes. Use of ELISA and similar methods to investigate predictive markers of graft dysfunction during cold ischemia is limited by the time needed to perform an assay. Rapid RT-PCR is an established technology that has potential for assessing predictive markers within a clinically relevant timeframe. With current knowledge of lung biology, the examination of cytokines has been a logical first step in looking for predictive markers of donor lung function. The biology of lung transplantation is not completely understood, however, and other predictive markers may exist in pathways not currently believed involved in graft failure or in novel pathways. To that end, two studies have used gene array technology and pathway analysis in an attempt to find novel markers of graft failure. Ray and colleagues[53] compared the expression profile of genes in PGD lungs and non-PGD lungs. A resulting 23 up-regulated and 42 down-regulated genes were identified but many of these differentially expressed transcripts had no known function. Anraku and colleagues[54] furthered the use of gene array analysis in donor lung evaluation by identifying four significantly up-regulated genes in a case-control study of PGD versus non-PGD patients and then verifying their predictive ability in a test set of 81 patients. This powerful combination of identifying predictive markers using gene chips, coupled with rapid RT-PCR to test these markers in a clinically relevant timeframe, likely will play a large role in the future of donor lung assessment.

EX VIVO ASSESSMENT

Although biomarkers may improve the organ selection process, lung function and lung physiology remain important parameters in lung assessment. Currently, the evaluation process is performed before and during the lung retrieval operation. This occurs, however, with the lung functioning within the perturbed physiologic environment of a brain-dead donor. EVLP is a new technique that allows for careful visual inspection of the explanted lungs, hemodynamic and ventilatory measurements, and evaluation of gas exchange. The set-up used in Leuven and elsewhere for the evaluation of human lungs declined for primary transplantation is similar to the circuit pioneered by Steen.[6,55-57] The closed circuit contains a blood reservoir, a centrifugal pump, a leukocyte filter, a gas exchanger, an inline blood gas analyzer, and a heater/cooler. An endotracheal tube and perfusion cannulas are inserted for inflow of venous blood through the pulmonary artery and outflow of saturated blood from the left atrium before the human double lung block is mounted in a Plexiglas box. Full perfusion of the lungs at a perfusion pressure less than or equal to 20 mm Hg is done at 37°C with Steen Solution (Vitrolife, Gothenburg, Sweden) mixed with a red blood cell concentrate up to a haematocrit of 15%. Functional assessment is performed during a period of 2 hours with measurement of gas exchange, hemodynamic and aerodynamic parameters, and indicators of lung edema.

EVLP is advantageous because (1) the ex vivo system provides an excellent environment for recruitment and re-expansion of atelectatic lung areas; (2) it allows for effective bronchial cleaning of secretions; (3) it allows for removal of clots in the pulmonary circulation through the use of transient retrograde perfusion at the beginning of the procedure, and (4) it allows for all ventilatory volumes and pressures to be transferred directly to the lungs without interference by the immobile chest wall and diaphragm, thereby improving ventilation/perfusion matching. Efforts with EVLP failed in the past largely because of tissue edema. Previous attempts at isolated organ perfusion at normothermic temperatures using acellular solutions have resulted in deteriorating perfusion characteristics and metabolic function after relatively short periods.[58,59] It is apparent that previous attempts at mimicking in vivo physiology in an ex vivo perfusion circuit failed for two major reasons. First, failure to maintain the integrity and normal barrier functions of the vasculature and epithelial beds led to a rapid deterioration in vascular flow and the concurrent development of edema. Secondly, the inability to support adequate delivery of nutrients and oxygen led to a deteriorating metabolic state. The modern success of EVLP without edema formation is in part the result of use of a buffered, extracellular solution with an optimal colloid osmotic pressure as the lung perfusate developed by Steen and colleagues,[55] sold commercially as Steen Solution. Steen's group has used a normothermic ex vivo circuit for evaluation of pig and human NHBDs with successful subsequent clinical transplantation and survival.[6,55] Neyrinck and colleagues[57] has reported a feasibility study with ex vivo reperfusion of 20 paired human lungs from DNDD donors. Other groups also have published their experience using a similar ex vivo reperfusion set-up.[56,60]

With the success of short-term ex vivo evaluation, extension of normothermic ex vivo perfusion beyond the short timeframe needed for evaluation only and into the longer timeframe needed for preservation or repair of poorly functioning lungs has been a highly topical area of active research. Erasmus and colleagues[61] extended ex vivo preservation to 6 hours in a pig model as part of a study to evaluate two different clinical NHBD protocols. They found that there was no development of lung edema; however, there was a statistically significant increase in pulmonary vascular resistance and maximum ventilation pressure at the end of 6 hours. This points to lung injury induced by the perfusion circuit itself occurring over the 6 hours of perfusion. Cypel and colleagues[62] in Toronto have subsequently developed an ex vivo circuit and perfusion and ventilation strategy, which can allow for successful 12-hour normothermic ex vivo perfusion without inducing edema and with stable pulmonary vascular resistance, airway pressures, and lung oxygenation capacity (**Fig. 1**). An acellular perfusate and a stable positive left atrial pressure (3–5 mm Hg) were two factors that helped to achieve this aim.[63] Stable perfusion for 12 hours under normothermic conditions would allow for ex vivo assessment, treatment, and even more sophisticated pharmacologic or molecular therapeutic repair of injured donor lungs.

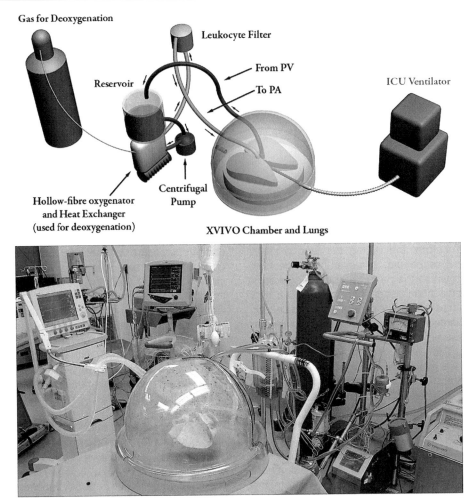

Fig. 1. Schematic of ex vivo perfusion circuit. The lungs are placed within the XVIVO chamber (Vitrolife, Gothenburg, Sweden). A cannula with pressure monitoring lines is sewn onto the pulmonary artery (PA) and another onto the left atrium. Using Steen Solution as a perfusate, a retrograde flush is performed and then the lungs are perfused anterograde. The perfusate leaves the lungs via the left atrial cannula and enters the reservoir. From there, the perfusate is pumped using a centrifugal pump into the oxygenator and heat exchanger where it is deoxygenated by a gas mixture (86% N_2, 8% CO_2, and 6% O_2) and heated to normothermia. The perfusate then passes through a leukocyte filter before reentering the lungs via the pulmonary artery cannula for oxygenation. PV, pulmonary vein.

RESUSCITATION STRATEGIES

Strategies to resuscitate donor lungs occur in vivo as part of donor management.[64,65] Physiologic changes after brain death are extremely deleterious to all potential donor organs and cardiovascular, endocrine, respiratory, and renal disturbances all contribute to organ demise.[66] Fortunately, careful and aggressive donor management has helped increase organ recovery and has been shown to improve P/F ratio from initial brain death to organ retrieval.[39,65,67]

The catecholamine storm during brain death can cause neurogenic pulmonary edema from the sudden and profound increase in systemic vascular resistance (SVR) leading to equally sudden increases in left atrial pressure and pulmonary capillary pressure.[68] After herniation and formal brain death, catecholamine levels drop and hypotension persists.[49,69] This hypotension is multifactorial and includes factors, such as vasomotor center death, causing decreased SVR, left heart dysfunction, and hypovolemia from diabetes insipidus and diuretic use for increased intracranial pressure before brain death.[70] To avoid aggravating neurogenic pulmonary edema and to avoid edema from hypervolemia, care to maintain euvolemia in donors is paramount. All potential donors should have central venous pressure (CVP) monitoring to maintain a CVP of between 4 and 10 mm Hg.[71] A pulmonary artery catheter should be considered for wedge pressure measurements when left heart dysfunction is suspected as CVP may be misleadingly low. If needed, dopamine (<10 ug/kg/min) and vasopressin (<2.4 U/h) are preferred vasopressors as first and second choices, respectively,[72] because norepinephrine and epinephrine are associated with lung dysfunction.[73,74] Vasopressin infusion has the added benefit of improving hypotension as a result not only of its vasopressor action but also its antidiuretic hormone action when diabetes insipidus is present.[75–77] It should be titrated to a SVR of 800 to 1200 $dyn \cdot s \cdot cm^5$ when a pulmonary artery catheter is present.[3]

Protective lung ventilation strategies similar to the strategy for acute respiratory distress syndrome (tidal volume = 6–8 mL/kg, PEEP = 5 mm Hg, $F_{IO_2} < .5$) should be used. A methylprednisolone bolus at 15 mg/kg has been shown to improve lung function and post-transplant outcomes.[67,78] It is unclear whether or not this is a result of the anti-inflammatory effect or a result of steroid replacement in the setting of corticotropin deficiency after brain death.

Lungs also are directly susceptible to atelectasis and pneumonia, in particular ventilator-associated pneumonia. Frequent turning and suctioning for pulmonary toilet is important. Regular recruitment maneuvers should be performed to avoid atelectasis. Bronchoscopy for removal of mucous plugs and bronchoalveolar lavage specimens for cultures also should be performed. Serial chest radiographs should be obtained to monitor any possible infiltrates.[3,39,72]

Angel and colleagues[65] recently have used retrospective data to show the impact of a standardized donor management protocol on resuscitating poor quality donors. In the 4-year period after initiation of their protocol, of 254 donors initially classified as "poor," 135 were able to be reclassified as "extended" or' ideal" at the end of donor management. Ultimately, 21% of donors originally classified as "poor" were used for lung transplantation. In comparison, before the initiation of the standardized donor protocol, only 10% of lungs were used from donors originally classified as "poor." Gabbay and colleagues[39] also have had success with improving P/F ratio with a donor management strategy. Of 140 consecutive transplants, 20 donors who originally would have been rejected were used successfully without impact on 30-day and 3-year survival rates. Others also have shown increased yield with active donor management.[64,67,79]

EX VIVO RESUSCITATION

In vivo donor management is important to mitigate the effects of brain death physiology. Despite the best medical management of donors, however, the donor lungs remain in the hostile environment of aberrant brain death physiology. Most donor management strategies aim to prevent further damage rather than produce or allow repair. Futhermore, organ retrieval often has to occur before the lungs have time to recover from brain death–related or other injury. With stable, noninjurious, 12-hour normothermic ex vivo perfusion now possible, repair of lungs ex vivo is a promising new strategy for assessment and repair of donor lungs. Possible pharmacologic applications of this circuit include using high osmotic perfusates or β-adrenergic drugs[80] to accelerate removal of lung edema, perfusing the lung with high-dose antibiotics to help sterilize pneumonias, and using fibrinolytics to help remove pulmonary emboli.

EX VIVO GENE THERAPY FOR LUNG REPAIR

One exciting method of lung repair is using gene therapy.[81] Gene therapy in lung transplantation is attractive because transtracheal delivery of gene vectors can localize the effect to the lung graft. In addition, the time point for a target of gene therapy—before reperfusion—is predictable. Up-regulation of the gene of interest need be present only at that specific time. Difficulties with lifelong gene expression, such as that needed in treating diseases, including cystic fibrosis, are not relevant in this scenario. Many target genes have been studied in gene therapy for lung transplantation. Antagonists of inflammatory mediators, such as soluble TNF receptor or soluble IL-1 receptor, to reduce ischemia-reperfusion injury are possibilities.[82,83] Interfering with T-cell activation by up-regulating CTLA4Ig and CD40Ig to reduce acute rejection are other options.[84,85] Gene therapy also provides the potential to immunologically pre-prepare donor lungs before exposure to the recipient immune system response.

In Toronto, gene transfer–mediated IL-10 up-regulation to reduce ischemia-reperfusion injury has been studied and will be discussed as an example of the concept of ex vivo gene therapy in donor lungs in this article. Severe ischemia-reperfusion injury remains a major cause of primary graft failure and early death. Levels of the proinflammatory cytokine IL-8 and the ratio of IL-6 to IL-10 have been shown to correlate with early graft failure.[50–52]

IL-10 is an anti-inflammatory cytokine that can limit the inflammatory and immune response.[86–88] Initial interest in the clinical use of recombinant IL-10 has been limited by its short half-life, systemic distribution, and high cost.[89,90] Thus, a gene therapy approach to introduce IL-10 to donor lungs has been studied.[91–98] An attractive gene vector in this setting is the adenoviral vector. It can be produced in quantities needed for transduction of a human or large animal lung; gene transfer occurs epichromosomally so insertional mutagenesis is not a concern, and it can transfect terminally differentiated cells.[81,99] In recent studies, adenovirus-mediated transfer of human IL-10 in vivo has been shown to reduce reperfusion injury in small and large animals.[91,96] The inflammatory reaction after in vivo administration of an adenovirus, however, although controllable, is still present and related primarily to activation of the innate immune response.[100] High-dose steroids have been found useful in dampening the immune response, but at least 6 hours is needed after transduction to have adequate gene expression.[95] Thus, ex vivo gene transfer may be more attractive because of the separation of the lung from the host immune system and the aberrant physiology of brain death. Logistically, ex vivo transduction is more convenient as it does not need to take place in an ICU at a distant hospital, eliminating delays in retrieval of other organs. Current cold static preservation limits the metabolic rate to the point that ex vivo transfected lungs do not express the transduced gene until after reperfusion.[63] Using normothermic EVLP, ex vivo transduction has been shown to be possible with gene expression occurring during perfusion. Cypel and colleagues[62,63] transfected pig lungs on EVLP using adenovirus encoding IL-10 for 12 h and showed superior lung function 4 h after transplantation after 12 h of cold ischemia. Human lungs rejected clinically for transplantation then were transfected and showed superior lung function and structural repair after 12 hours of EVLP.[101] This study is an important proof of concept for ex vivo gene therapy using prolonged EVLP as a platform and represents a powerful and promising method of donor lung repair.

SUMMARY

The shortage of adequate organ donors remains a great challenge in clinical lung transplantation. With increasing experience in the medical management and surgical technique of lung transplantation, gradual expansion of the criteria for lung donor selection has occurred with beneficial effects on the donor pool. Interest in donation after cardiac death also is increasing as the gap increases between donors and the needs of listed patients. Successful use of these new sources of lungs depends on the accurate assessment and prediction of transplanted lung function. Promising techniques for lung assessment and diagnostics include investigating key genes associated with graft failure or good graft performance using molecular approaches, and ex vivo evaluation. Further studies are needed to answer remaining questions about the best technique and solution to reperfuse human lungs for several hours without edema formation. As the predictive ability to discern good from injured donor lungs improves, strategies to repair donor lungs become increasingly important. Prolonged normothermic EVLP seems to be a platform on which many reparative strategies can be realized. With these new methods for assessing and resuscitating lungs accurately, it is hoped that inroads will be made toward providing every listed patient a chance for successful lung transplantation.

ACKNOWLEDGMENTS

Shaf Keshavjee and Thomas K. Waddell are supported by Canadian Institutes of Health Research grants. Jonathan C. Yeung is supported by the Surgeon Scientist Program at the University of Toronto. Dirk van Raemdonck is supported by grant OT/03/55 from Katholieke Universiteit Leuven and by grant G.3C04.99 from the Fund for Scientific Research—Flanders.

REFERENCES

1. Trulock EP, Christie JD, Edwards LB, et al. Registry of the International Society for Heart and Lung Transplantation: twenty-fourth official adult lung and heart-lung transplantation report—2007. J Heart Lung Transplant 2007;26(8):782–95.
2. Reports UNfOSD. National Data. 2008. Available at: http://www.unos.org/data/about/viewDataReports.asp. Accessed June 24, 2008.
3. de Perrot M, Weder W, Patterson GA, et al. Strategies to increase limited donor resources. Eur Respir J 2004;23(3):477–82.
4. Kootstra G, Kievit J, Nederstigt A. Organ donors: heartbeating and non-heartbeating. World J Surg 2002;26(2):181–4.
5. Steinbrook R. Organ donation after cardiac death. N Engl J Med 2007;357(3):209–13.
6. Steen S, Sjoberg T, Pierre L, et al. Transplantation of lungs from a non-heart-beating donor. Lancet 2001; 357(9259):825–9.
7. Orens JB, Boehler A, de Perrot M, et al. A review of lung transplant donor acceptability criteria. J Heart Lung Transplant 2003;22(11):1183–200.

8. Arcasoy SM, Fisher A, Hachem RR, et al. Report of the ISHLT Working Group on primary lung graft dysfunction part V: predictors and outcomes. J Heart Lung Transplant 2005;24(10):1483–8.

9. Ware LB, Wang Y, Fang X, et al. Assessment of lungs rejected for transplantation and implications for donor selection. Lancet 2002;360(9333):619–20.

10. Kootstra G, Daemen JH, Oomen AP. Categories of non-heart-beating donors. Transplant Proc 1995; 27(5):2893–4.

11. Hardy JD, Webb WR, Dalton ML Jr, et al. Lung homotransplantation in man. JAMA 1963;186: 1065–74.

12. A definition of irreversible coma. Report of the Ad Hoc Committee of the Harvard Medical School to Examine the Definition of Brain Death. JAMA 1968;205(6):337–40.

13. Egan TM, Lambert CJ Jr, Reddick R, et al. A strategy to increase the donor pool: use of cadaver lungs for transplantation. Ann Thorac Surg 1991; 52(5):1113–20 [discussion: 1120–1].

14. Ulicny KS Jr, Egan TM, Lambert CJ Jr. Cadaver lung donors: effect of preharvest ventilation on graft function. Ann Thorac Surg 1993;55(5): 1185–91.

15. Alessandrini F, D'Armini AM, Roberts CS, et al. When does the lung die? II. Ultrastructural evidence of pulmonary viability after "death". J Heart Lung Transplant 1994;13(5):748–57.

16. D'Armini AM, Roberts CS, Griffith PK, et al. When does the lung die? I. Histochemical evidence of pulmonary viability after "death". J Heart Lung Transplant 1994;13(5):741–7.

17. Egan TM. Non-heart-beating donors in thoracic transplantation. J Heart Lung Transplant 2004; 23(1):3–10.

18. Van Raemdonck DE, Rega FR, Neyrinck AP, et al. Non-heart-beating donors. Semin Thorac Cardiovasc Surg 2004;16(4):309–21.

19. Love RB, Stringham J, Chomiak PN, et al. First successful lung transplantation using a nonheart-beating donor. J Heart Lung Transplant 1995; 14(S):S88.

20. Love RB, D'Allesandro AM, Cornwell RA, et al. Ten year experience with human lung transplantation from non-heart beating donors. J Heart Lung Transplant 2003;22(1 Suppl 1):S87.

21. Nunez JR, Varela A, del Rio F, et al. Bipulmonary transplants with lungs obtained from two non-heart-beating donors who died out of hospital. J Thorac Cardiovasc Surg 2004;127(1):297–9.

22. Gamez P, Cordoba M, Ussetti P, et al. Lung transplantation from out-of-hospital non-heart-beating lung donors. one-year experience and results. J Heart Lung Transplant 2005;24(8):1098–102.

23. de Antonio DG, Marcos R, Laporta R, et al. Results of clinical lung transplant from uncontrolled non-heart-beating donors. J Heart Lung Transplant 2007;26(5):529–34.

24. Erasmus ME, van der Bij W, Verschuuren EAM. 56: non-heart-beating lung donation in the Netherlands: the first experience. J Heart Lung Transplant 2006;25(2 Suppl 1):S63.

25. Butt TA, Aitchison JD, Corris PA, et al. 140: lung transplantation from deceased donors without pretreatment. J Heart Lung Transplant 2007; 26(2, Suppl 1):S110.

26. Oto T, Levvey B, McEgan R, et al. A practical approach to clinical lung transplantation from a Maastricht Category III donor with cardiac death. J Heart Lung Transplant 2007;26(2):196–9.

27. Van Raemdonck D, Verleden GM, Dupont L, et al. 382: initial experience with lung transplantation from non-heart-beating donors. J Heart Lung Transplant 2008;27(2, Suppl 1):S198–9.

28. Steen S, Ingemansson R, Budrikis A, et al. Successful transplantation of lungs topically cooled in the non-heart-beating donor for 6 hours. Ann Thorac Surg 1997;63(2):345–51.

29. Rega FR, Neyrinck AP, Verleden GM, et al. How long can we preserve the pulmonary graft inside the nonheart-beating donor? Ann Thorac Surg 2004;77(2):438–44 [discussion: 444].

30. Steen S, Ingemansson R, Eriksson L, et al. First human transplantation of a nonacceptable donor lung after reconditioning ex vivo. Ann Thorac Surg 2007;83(6):2191–4.

31. Van Raemdonck DE, Jannis NC, De Leyn PR, et al. Warm ischemic tolerance in collapsed pulmonary grafts is limited to 1 hour. Ann Surg 1998;228(6): 788–96.

32. Snell GI, Levvey BJ, Williams TJ. Non-heart beating organ donation. Intern Med J 2004;34(8):501–3.

33. Aigner C, Seebacher G, Klepetko W. Lung transplantation. Donor selection. Chest Surg Clin N Am 2003;13(3):429–42.

34. Van De Wauwer C, Neyrinck A, Geudens N, et al. The mode of death in the non-heart-beating donor has an impact on lung graft quality. Interact Cardiovasc Thorac Surg 2007;6(S2):199.

35. Sohrabi S, Navarro A, Asher J, et al. Agonal period in potential non-heart-beating donors. Transplant Proc 2006;38(8):2629–30.

36. Snell GI, Griffiths A, Levvey BJ, et al. Availability of lungs for transplantation: exploring the real potential of the donor pool. J Heart Lung Transplant 2008;27(6):662–7.

37. Bhorade SM, Vigneswaran W, McCabe MA, et al. Liberalization of donor criteria may expand the donor pool without adverse consequence in lung transplantation. J Heart Lung Transplant 2000; 19(12):1199–204.

38. Botha P, Trivedi D, Weir CJ, et al. Extended donor criteria in lung transplantation: impact on organ

allocation. J Thorac Cardiovasc Surg 2006;131(5): 1154–60.

39. Gabbay E, Williams TJ, Griffiths AP, et al. Maximizing the utilization of donor organs offered for lung transplantation. Am J Respir Crit Care Med 1999;160(1):265–71.

40. Kron IL, Tribble CG, Kern JA, et al. Successful transplantation of marginally acceptable thoracic organs. Ann Surg 1993;217(5):518–22 [discussion: 522–4].

41. Lardinois D, Banysch M, Korom S, et al. Extended donor lungs: eleven years experience in a consecutive series. Eur J Cardiothorac Surg 2005;27(5): 762–7.

42. Pierre AF, Sekine Y, Hutcheon MA, et al. Marginal donor lungs: a reassessment. J Thorac Cardiovasc Surg 2002;123(3):421–7 [discussion: 427–8].

43. Sundaresan S, Semenkovich J, Ochoa L, et al. Successful outcome of lung transplantation is not compromised by the use of marginal donor lungs. J Thorac Cardiovasc Surg 1995;109(6):1075–9 [discussion: 1079–80].

44. Oto T, Levvey BJ, Whitford H, et al. Feasibility and utility of a lung donor score: correlation with early post-transplant outcomes. Ann Thorac Surg 2007; 83(1):257–63.

45. Cypel M, Yildirim E, Boasquevisque C, et al. Donor scoring does not predict early outcome. J Heart Lung Transplant 2008;27(2):S251.

46. de Perrot M, Liu M, Waddell TK, et al. Ischemia-reperfusion-induced lung injury. Am J Respir Crit Care Med 2003;167(4):490–511.

47. Amado JA, Lopez-Espadas F, Vazquez-Barquero A, et al. Blood levels of cytokines in brain-dead patients: relationship with circulating hormones and acute-phase reactants. Metabolism 1995; 44(6):812–6.

48. Avlonitis VS, Fisher AJ, Kirby JA, et al. Pulmonary transplantation: the role of brain death in donor lung injury. Transplantation 2003;75(12):1928–33.

49. Pratschke J, Wilhelm MJ, Kusaka M, et al. Brain death and its influence on donor organ quality and outcome after transplantation. Transplantation 1999;67(3):343–8.

50. de Perrot M, Sekine Y, Fischer S, et al. Interleukin-8 release during early reperfusion predicts graft function in human lung transplantation. Am J Respir Crit Care Med 2002;165(2):211–5.

51. Fisher AJ, Donnelly SC, Hirani N, et al. Elevated levels of interleukin-8 in donor lungs is associated with early graft failure after lung transplantation. Am J Respir Crit Care Med 2001;163(1):259–65.

52. Kaneda H, Waddell TK, de Perrot M, et al. Pre-implantation multiple cytokine mRNA expression analysis of donor lung grafts predicts survival after lung transplantation in humans. Am J Transplant 2006;6(3):544–51.

53. Ray M, Dharmarajan S, Freudenberg J, et al. Expression profiling of human donor lungs to understand primary graft dysfunction after lung transplantation. Am J Transplant 2007;7(10): 2396–405.

54. Anraku M, Cameron MJ, Waddell TK, et al. Impact of human donor lung gene expression profiles on survival after lung transplantation: a case-control study. Am J Transplant 2008;8(10):2140–8.

55. Steen S, Liao Q, Wierup PN, et al. Transplantation of lungs from non-heart-beating donors after functional assessment ex vivo. Ann Thorac Surg 2003; 76(1):244–52 [discussion: 252].

56. Wierup P, Haraldsson A, Nilsson F, et al. Ex vivo evaluation of nonacceptable donor lungs. Ann Thorac Surg 2006;81(2):460–6.

57. Neyrinck A, Rega F, Jannis N, et al. Ex vivo reperfusion of human lungs declined for transplantation; a novel approach to alleviate donor organ shortage? J Heart Lung Transplant 2004;23(2 Suppl 1):S172–3.

58. Brandes H, Albes JM, Conzelmann A, et al. Comparison of pulsatile and nonpulsatile perfusion of the lung in an extracorporeal large animal model. Eur Surg Res 2002;34(4):321–9.

59. Hardesty RL, Griffith BP. Autoperfusion of the heart and lungs for preservation during distant procurement. J Thorac Cardiovasc Surg 1987;93(1):11–8.

60. Egan TM, Haithcock JA, Nicotra WA, et al. Ex vivo evaluation of human lungs for transplant suitability. Ann Thorac Surg 2006;81(4):1205–13.

61. Erasmus ME, Fernhout MH, Elstrodt JM, et al. Normothermic ex vivo lung perfusion of non-heart-beating donor lungs in pigs: from pretransplant function analysis towards a 6-h machine preservation. Transpl Int 2006;19(7):589–93.

62. Cypel M, Yeung J, Hirayama S, et al. Technique for prolonged normothermic ex vivo lung perfusion. J Heart Lung Transplant 2008;27(12): 1319–25.

63. Cypel M, Hirayama S, Rubacha M, et al. 385: Ex-Vivo Normothermic Lung Perfusion (EVLP) interrupts ischemic injury and restores cellular metabolism. J Heart Lung Transplant 2008;27(2 Suppl 1): S199–200.

64. Straznicka M, Follette DM, Eisner MD, et al. Aggressive management of lung donors classified as unacceptable: excellent recipient survival one year after transplantation. J Thorac Cardiovasc Surg 2002;124(2):250–8.

65. Angel LF, Levine DJ, Restrepo MI, et al. Impact of a lung transplantation donor-management protocol on lung donation and recipient outcomes. Am J Respir Crit Care Med 2006;174(6):710–6.

66. Novitzky D. Detrimental effects of brain death on the potential organ donor. Transplant Proc 1997; 29(8):3770–2.

67. Venkateswaran RV, Patchell VB, Wilson IC, et al. Early donor management increases the retrieval rate of lungs for transplantation. Ann Thorac Surg 2008;85(1):278–86 [discussion: 286].

68. Novitzky D, Wicomb WN, Rose AG, et al. Pathophysiology of pulmonary edema following experimental brain death in the chacma baboon. Ann Thorac Surg 1987;43(3):288–94.

69. Marshall VC. Pathophysiology of brain death: effects on allograft function. Transplant Proc 2001; 33(1–2):845–6.

70. Linos K, Fraser J, Freeman WD, et al. Care of the brain-dead organ donor. Curr Anaesth Crit Care 2007;18(5–6):284–94.

71. Pennefather SH, Bullock RE, Dark JH. The effect of fluid therapy on alveolar arterial oxygen gradient in brain-dead organ donors. Transplantation 1993; 56(6):1418–22.

72. Shemie SD, Ross H, Pagliarello J, et al. Organ donor management in Canada: recommendations of the forum on medical management to optimize donor organ potential. CMAJ 2006;174(6):S13–32.

73. Schnuelle P, Berger S, de Boer J, et al. Effects of catecholamine application to brain-dead donors on graft survival in solid organ transplantation. Transplantation 2001;72(3):455–63.

74. Mukadam ME, Harrington DK, Wilson IC, et al. Does donor catecholamine administration affect early lung function after transplantation? J Thorac Cardiovasc Surg 2005;130(3):926–7.

75. Rostron AJ, Avlonitis VS, Cork DM, et al. Hemodynamic resuscitation with arginine vasopressin reduces lung injury after brain death in the transplant donor. Transplantation 2008;85(4):597–606.

76. Pennefather SH, Bullock RE, Mantle D, et al. Use of low dose arginine vasopressin to support brain-dead organ donors. Transplantation 1995;59(1): 58–62.

77. Debaveye YA, Van den Berghe GH. Is there still a place for dopamine in the modern intensive care unit? Anesth Analg 2004;98(2):461–8.

78. Follette DM, Rudich SM, Babcock WD. Improved oxygenation and increased lung donor recovery with high-dose steroid administration after brain death. J Heart Lung Transplant 1998;17(4):423–9.

79. Rosendale JD, Chabalewski FL, McBride MA, et al. Increased transplanted organs from the use of a standardized donor management protocol. Am J Transplant 2002;2(8):761–8.

80. Ware LB, Fang X, Wang Y, et al. Selected contribution: mechanisms that may stimulate the resolution of alveolar edema in the transplanted human lung. J Appl Physiol 2002;93(5):1869–74.

81. Sato M, Keshavjee S. Gene therapy in lung transplantation. Curr Gene Ther 2006;6(4):439–58.

82. Tagawa T, Kozower BD, Kanaan SA, et al. Tumor necrosis factor inhibitor gene transfer ameliorates

lung graft ischemia-reperfusion injury. J Thorac Cardiovasc Surg 2003;126(4):1147–54.

83. Tagawa T, Dharmarajan S, Hayama M, et al. Endobronchial gene transfer of soluble type I interleukin-1 receptor ameliorates lung graft ischemia-reperfusion injury. Ann Thorac Surg 2004;78(6): 1932–9 [discussion: 1939].

84. Ugurlu MM, Griffin MD, O'Brien T, et al. The effects of CTLA-4Ig on acute lung allograft rejection: a comparison of intrabronchial gene therapy with systemic administration of protein. Transplantation 2001;71(12):1867–71.

85. Chang GJ, Liu T, Feng S, et al. Targeted gene therapy with CD40Ig to induce long-term acceptance of liver allografts. Surgery 2002;132(2): 149–56.

86. de Waal Malefyt R, Haanen J, Spits H, et al. Interleukin 10 (IL-10) and viral IL-10 strongly reduce antigen-specific human T cell proliferation by diminishing the antigen-presenting capacity of monocytes via downregulation of class II major histocompatibility complex expression. J Exp Med 1991;174(4):915–24.

87. Fiorentino DF, Bond MW, Mosmann TR. Two types of mouse T helper cell. IV. Th2 clones secrete a factor that inhibits cytokine production by Th1 clones. J Exp Med 1989;170(6):2081–95.

88. Moore KW, de Waal Malefyt R, Coffman RL, et al. Interleukin-10 and the interleukin-10 receptor. Annu Rev Immunol 2001;19:683–765.

89. Asadullah K, Sterry W, Volk HD. Interleukin-10 therapy—review of a new approach. Pharmacol Rev 2003;55(2):241–69.

90. Eppinger MJ, Ward PA, Bolling SF, et al. Regulatory effects of interleukin-10 on lung ischemia-reperfusion injury. J Thorac Cardiovasc Surg 1996; 112(5):1301–5 [discussion: 1305–6].

91. Fischer S, Liu M, MacLean AA, et al. In vivo transtracheal adenovirus-mediated transfer of human interleukin-10 gene to donor lungs ameliorates ischemia-reperfusion injury and improves early posttransplant graft function in the rat. Hum Gene Ther 2001;12(12):1513–26.

92. Itano H, Mora BN, Zhang W, et al. Lipid-mediated ex vivo gene transfer of viral interleukin 10 in rat lung allotransplantation. J Thorac Cardiovasc Surg 2001;122(1):29–38.

93. Itano H, Zhang W, Ritter JH, et al. Adenovirus-mediated gene transfer of human interleukin 10 ameliorates reperfusion injury of rat lung isografts. J Thorac Cardiovasc Surg 2000;120(5):947–56.

94. Itano H, Zhang W, Ritter JH, et al. Endobronchial transfection of naked viral interleukin-10 gene in rat lung allotransplantation. Ann Thorac Surg 2001;71(4):1126–33.

95. de Perrot M, Fischer S, Liu M, et al. Impact of human interleukin-10 on vector-induced

inflammation and early graft function in rat lung transplantation. Am J Respir Cell Mol Biol 2003; 28(5):616–25.

96. Martins S, de Perrot M, Imai Y, et al. Transbronchial administration of adenoviral-mediated interleukin-10 gene to the donor improves function in a pig lung transplant model. Gene Ther 2004;11(24):1786–96.

97. Kanaan SA, Kozower BD, Suda T, et al. Intratracheal adenovirus-mediated gene transfer is optimal in experimental lung transplantation. J Thorac Cardiovasc Surg 2002;124(6):1130–6.

98. Kozower BD, Kanaan SA, Tagawa T, et al. Intramuscular gene transfer of interleukin-10 reduces neutrophil recruitment and ameliorates lung graft ischemia-reperfusion injury. Am J Transplant 2002;2(9):837–42.

99. Romano G, Michell P, Pacilio C, et al. Latest developments in gene transfer technology: achievements, perspectives, and controversies over therapeutic applications. Stem Cells 2000;18(1):19–39.

100. Zsengeller ZK, Wert SE, Hull WM, et al. Persistence of replication-deficient adenovirus-mediated gene transfer in lungs of immune-deficient (nu/nu) mice. Hum Gene Ther 1995;6(4):457–67.

101. Cypel M, Rubacha M, Hirayama S, et al. 331: ex-vivo repair and regeneration of damaged human donor lungs. J Heart Lung Transplant 2008;27(2 Suppl 1):S180.

Update on Lung Transplantation for Emphysema

Chadrick E. Denlinger, MD, Bryan F. Meyers, MD, MPH*

KEYWORDS

- Lung transplantation • Adverse effects • Emphysema
- Obstructive lung disease • Patient selection
- Statistics and numerical data

Significant improvements in human lung transplantation have occurred since the first successful single lung transplant in 1983 and the first bilateral transplant in 1986. The annual number of lung transplants continues to rise slowly with recent data reported by the International Society for Heart and Lung Transplantation (ISHLT) showing 2196 single and bilateral transplants in 2005.[1] Despite improvements with donor selection, challenges remain in lung preservation, recipient prioritization, perioperative mortality, and long-term morbidity. In an effort to optimize the benefits derived from lung transplantation, the United Network for Organ Sharing (UNOS) recently reorganized the prioritization scheme by which potential recipients were listed. The focus of this article is to review the current status of lung transplantation for emphysema, with attention given to current outcomes and management strategies.

DONOR SELECTION

Donor lung quality is one the most important factors contributing to the early perioperative success of lung transplants. Ideal donors as defined by the ISHLT are patients less than or equal to 50 years old, less than or equal to 20 pack-year smoking history, and pO_2 greater than 300 mmHg with a 100% FiO_2 oxygen challenge without pulmonary infiltrates on a chest radiograph. In addition, the location of the donor should be within a reasonable distance of the recipient institution to allow an ischemic time less than 6 hours. Although data suggests that each component defining an ideal donor can be individually challenged with acceptable results, common wisdom holds that the best outcomes will be achieved with lungs from an ideal donor. Further details relating to the selection of potential lung donors and optimization of organ procurement will be discussed thoroughly in other chapters of this publication.

RECIPIENT SELECTION

Recently, the relative frequencies of the common indications for lung transplantation have changed. It was once thought that emphysema represented an absolute contraindication for single lung transplantation because of perceived risks of ventilation/perfusion mismatches. However, emphysema has become the most common indication for lung transplantation, which is currently 33% to 36% of all transplants. Emphysema is followed closely by interstitial pulmonary fibrosis (IPF) at 24% to 33%, CF at 12% to 16%, and primary pulmonary hypertension (PPH) at 2% to 7%.[2,3] The average recipient age for contemporary transplants is 51.2 ($\pm$ 13.0) years, and transplants are equally distributed between men and women.[3] Corroborating data reported to the ISHLT continue to suggest that the most frequent indication for transplantation is COPD (38%) followed by IPF (19%), CF (16%) and α_1-antitrypsin deficiency emphysema (8%). Other rare indications accounting for less than 1% each of all lung transplants, are PPH, sarcoidosis, bronchiectasis, and lymphangioleiomatosis.

Department of Surgery, Washington University School of Medicine, 3108, Queeny Tower, One Barnes-Jewish Hospital Plaza, St. Louis, MO 63110-1013, USA
* Corresponding author.
E-mail address: meyersb@wustl.edu (B.F. Meyers).

Thorac Surg Clin 19 (2009) 275–283
doi:10.1016/j.thorsurg.2009.03.001

The decision to place a patient on the waiting list for a lung transplant is based primarily on the perceived likelihood that they will die without transplantation and that they are sufficiently healthy to live and thrive after transplantation. In the past, that determination was made locally by each individual center, but now those estimates are codified and summarized by a calculated lung allocation score (LAS) described below. In addition to the variables covered by the LAS, several other unsubstantiated factors contribute to the perioperative risks of the procedure such as prior thoracic surgery, chronic steroid use, and mechanical ventilation. Prior thoracic surgery, such as lung volume reduction surgery, increases the operative time and intraoperative blood loss, but has not been associated with worse overall survival outcomes.[4] Patients on chronic steroids have been considered to be at increased risk for bronchial dehiscence, but this concept was challenged by Park and colleagues. In this study, 26 subjects were studied after transplantation on chronic steroids with a doses ranging from 1.5 mg to 40 mg (mean 12.4 mg) of oral prednisone. None of the subjects suffered from a bronchial dehiscence. Incidentally, subjects taking steroids prior to transplant had a lower cumulative rate of airway anastomotic strictures at 3 years.[5]

Mechanical ventilation in patients with emphysema implies the final stages of their disease. Our group published a series of 21 lung transplants performed on subjects requiring preoperative ventilation. This subjects cohort was subdivided into stable subjects (n = 16) that were ventilated because of respiratory failure secondary to progression of their primary disease and unstable subjects (n = 5) suffering from primary graft dysfunction following an initial lung transplant. Three of the five unstable subjects died postoperatively but there were no postoperative deaths in the stable ventilated subjects. Expectedly, stable ventilated subjects had a longer postoperative intubation time, longer postoperative ICU stay, and longer overall hospital stay, but there was no significance difference in five-year survival when compared to nonventilated subjects receiving transplants in the same time frame.[6] These findings suggest that prior thoracic surgery, preoperative steroid risk, and ventilator dependence should not exclude patients from being listed for lung transplantation.

LUNG ALLOCATION SYSTEM

Historically, the most common indication for lung transplantation has been COPD because prior organ allocation schemes were based principally on the length of time patients spent on the transplant waiting list. Since the rate of disease progression is slower for COPD than for other diseases leading to transplantation, these patients were more likely to survive long enough to receive transplants. Ironically, these patients may also have derived the smallest gain from transplantation because of their relatively long expected survival with medical management. In 1995, a minor amendment to the seniority ranking list granted a 90-day bonus to patients with IPF when listed in an attempt to compensate for their expected higher wait-list mortality rate. However, in May 2005, UNOS completely replaced the seniority system with the LAS system that considers objective measures for disease severity, physiologic reserve and primary disease diagnosis to balance the medical urgency with the net expected time benefit of lung transplantation.

Revisions in the allocation system were driven, in part, by a growing list of patients on the waiting list and speculation that subsets of patients were being listed earlier than necessary in order to accrue waiting time in advance of actually needing a transplant. The increase in the number of patients on the waiting list correlated temporarily with a decreased mortality rate observed from greater than 200 per 1000 patient years in 1995 to 134 per 1000 patient years in 2004. This supports the concern that patients were prematurely listed in order to enhance the probability of receiving a transplant.[7]

The goal of the LAS system is to optimize the relative odds for 1-year survival with or without a lung transplant. A current exception to this prioritization scheme pertains to children less than 12 years old who remain prioritized based solely on the length of wait-list time. Patients less than 12 years old cannot currently be scored by the LAS system because insufficient survival data precludes accurate calculations for expected survival. Another exception to the LAS system involves lungs from donors aged 12 to 17 years that must be first offered to adolescents prioritized by the LAS score. If there are no appropriate recipients in this age range, these lungs are next offered to children aged less than 12 years before offering the lungs to the adult population.

The LAS is a composite number derived from a formula that takes into account factors from three principal categories. The first factor is the patient's primary pulmonary diagnosis. The second category relates to disease-specific factors objectifying the disease severity (pulmonary artery pressures, forced vital capacity, oxygen supplementation, and ventilator requirement). The third category addresses the overall patient health outside of their pulmonary disease, (age, BMI, New York Heart Association functional class, PCW, 6-minute walk distance, diabetes and serum creatinine). The UNOS calculator used to determine LAS scores can currently be found online at the following website: www.unos.org/resources/frm_LAS_Calculator.asp?index=98.[8] After determining LAS scores for individual patients, available lungs are allocated regionally according to a prioritized ranking based on LAS scores.

Early studies evaluating the effects of the new LAS scoring system on results have found that the total number of lung transplants performed in the United States have not changed.[9] A moderate redistribution of indications for transplant has been observed, where fewer patients with COPD received transplant while more patients with pulmonary fibrosis were transplanted.[1,3,9] The frequency of transplants for CF and PPH are virtually unchanged.[1] Thus, there was a shift favoring patients with the highest waiting list mortality rate. Since the implementation of the LAS system, the average time spent on the waiting list and the number of patients awaiting transplant have decreased. These findings are likely related to withdrawing patients from the active transplant waiting list who are either to sick for a transplant operation or who would have too low an LAS score to receive reasonable prioritization. As expected, the average LAS scores retrospectively calculated on patients transplanted prior to LAS implementation were significantly lower than more contemporary scores actually utilized for recipient prioritization. The mean LAS for patients receiving transplants after implementation of the scoring system was 42.5 ($\pm$ 15.2) compared to an average of 35.4 ($\pm$ 8.2) before introduction of the LAS system.[1]

Despite a shift toward transplanting patients with lower expected survival in the absence of transplantation, mortality rates after LAS implementation remain unchanged.[9] A large multi-institutional retrospective review of patients receiving lung transplants before and after the implementation of the LAS system showed that hospital mortality remained at 5.3% and that 1-year survival before and after LAS were 90% and 89% respectively.[3] Others found insignificant improvements in 1-year survival.[2] Variable results have also been reported for perioperative morbidity. Kozower and colleagues noted an increased incidence of primary graft dysfunction (14.1% versus 22.9%) and an increased ICU length of stay (5.7 versus 7.8 days) after LAS implementation.[3] Conversely, McCue reported that the ICU and hospital lengths of stay, time on the

ventilator, and primary graft dysfunction rates were unchanged.[2]

The principal objective of the LAS system was to reduce the waiting list mortality, though completion of such an objective is difficult to prove. Since LAS implementation, the mortality rate appears to have decreased from 15.3% to 11.3%, a decline that did not reach statistical significance in a moderately powered study ($P = .08$).[3] There is some concern, however, that changing wait-list mortality rates may relate to decisions made concerning which patients to list and when to list them. For example, a patient with COPD and a low LAS score may not be listed under the current system because the chances of receiving organs are low and there is no advantage gained by accruing time on the waiting list. These patients may remain off the waiting list and they will live or die without being recorded as a wait-list mortality. On the other hand, many high-risk patients are now listed, since their clinical condition translates into an LAS score that would offer hope of transplant in this system, but not the previous scheme. Therefore, with multiple changes in the decisions about listing, it remains unclear whether a decline in the waiting list mortality actually translates into a decreased mortality rate among all patients with end-stage pulmonary disease.

OUTCOMES

Benchmark survival rates by the ISHLT following lung transplantation are 87% at 3 months, 78% at 1 year, 62% at 3 years, and 50% at 5 years.[1] Survival for single- and double-transplant recipients are similar in the first postoperative year, but survival after bilateral transplant is superior in the subsequent years. When evaluating the two most recent 5-year time frames, 1-year survival has improved from 74% to 81%, and the 5-year survival has improved from 47% to 52%.

Long-term survival is better for patients transplanted for CF, α_1-antitrypsin deficiency, and PPH compared to either COPD or idiopathic pulmonary fibrosis.[1] This finding likely relates to differing ages and comorbidities among patients from different diagnosis groups. Patients receiving bilateral transplants had improved survival relative to single-lung transplants when performed for COPD, idiopathic pulmonary fibrosis or α_1-antitrypsin. The CMV status of recipients had no influence on long-term survival; whereas the survival of patients receiving organs from CMV-negative donors was better than from CMV-positive donors.

The intuitive advantages of lung transplantation include a complete replacement of the diseased and poorly functioning lungs with new and healthy donor lungs. Initial and long-term function of patients with single- or bilateral-lung transplants for emphysema shows a dramatic improvement in pulmonary function and exercise tolerance with elimination of the need for supplementary oxygen even when compared to lung volume reduction surgery.[10] **Fig. 1** demonstrates the magnitude of change in the FEV_1 as a result of single-lung transplantation, bilateral-lung transplantation, and lung volume reduction surgery as reported by Gaissert and colleagues. **Fig. 2** shows a similar stratified analysis for exercise tolerance measured by 6-minute walking distances. Although the improvement in both outcome measures is greatest for BLT and least for LVRS, the absolute differences in exercise tolerance are much less than those seen in pulmonary function.

The relative disadvantages of lung transplant for emphysema are worth reviewing. First, the lack of available donor lungs created a situation in which the waiting times for transplant recipients in many programs exceeded 2 years prior to implementation to the LAS system. The waiting times on the transplant list have decreased significantly; however, the current volume of lung transplants performed in the United States remains limited by the availability of donor lungs. Most patients with emphysema have a stability that is reflected in the lower LAS, and thus less likelihood of obtaining donor lungs. If and when lungs become available, the initial morbidity and mortality of a lung transplant are higher than that reported for lung volume reduction, with mortality variously

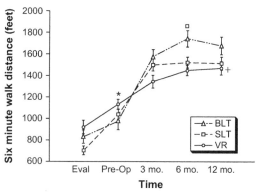

Fig. 2. Comparison of 6-minute walk distance before and after volume reduction (VR), single lung transplantation (SLT), and BLT. At evaluation (*): VR versus SLT, not significant; VR versus BLT, $P < .05$. At 6 months (□), VR versus SLT, not significant; VR versus BLT, $P < .001$. (+) VR Eval versus VR 6 mo, $P < .001$. (*From* Gaissert HA, Trulock EP, Cooper JD, et al. Comparison of early functional results after volume reduction or lung transplantation for chronic obstructive pulmonary disease. J Thorac Cardiovasc Surg 1996;111:302; with permission.)

described as 5% to 15% for the first 30 days and somewhat higher by the end of the first year. For the survivors, the presence of allograft lungs creates the need for lifelong immunosuppression that carries with it higher medical costs to the individual and society and an increased risk of neoplasm and infection when compared with nonimmunosuppressed patients. Finally, the risk of developing chronic allograft dysfunction, or bronchiolitis obliterans syndrome (BOS), increases as a function of time since transplant reaches 50% to 60% by 5 years after transplant. The cumulative 5-year survival of the authors' lung transplant experience is 50%, a fact that clearly demonstrates the imperfect solution that lung transplantation offers.

A controversial aspect of lung transplantation concerns the question of whether a survival benefit is conveyed to the recipient. There have been no prospective randomized trials in which lung transplantation has been directly compared to medical therapy as a treatment for advanced lung disease. In addition, the survival benefits afforded by this operation likely depend, in part, on the specific etiology of the lung disease. Survival following lung transplantation for COPD is comparable to survival following lung volume reduction.[10] As a result, the analysis of this question has been limited to the use of Cox regression analysis with the transplant procedure entered into the model as a time-dependent covariable. In essence, the patient's time spent on the waiting list is used as the medical arm of the trial, and the survival after

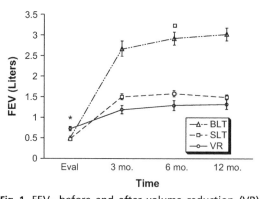

Fig. 1. FEV_1 before and after volume reduction (VR) single lung transplantation (SLT) and BLT. At evaluation (*): VR versus SLT, $P < .001$; VR versus BLT, $P < .001$. At 6 months (□), VR versus SLT, $P < .001$; VR versus BLT, $P < .001$. (+) VR Eval versus VR 6 mo, $P < .001$. (*From* Gaissert HA, Trulock EP, Cooper JD, et al. Comparison of early functional results after volume reduction or lung transplantation for chronic obstructive pulmonary disease. J Thorac Cardiovasc Surg 1996;111:300; with permission.)

transplantation is used as the surgical arm. One such analysis by Hosenpud and colleagues found that lung transplantation did not reduce the risk of death compared to the risks of the natural course of disease progression.[11] One explanation for this finding is that this study was conducted in an era prior to the implementation of the LAS scoring system, when patients on the waiting list with COPD were prematurely listed to accrue time. Other Cox regression models addressing the question of whether lung transplant conveys a survival benefit have shown clear survival benefit for patients with emphysema undergoing lung transplantation.[12]

The choice of bilateral or unilateral transplantation for patients with emphysema is controversial. Historically, single-lung transplants were frequently performed for patients diagnosed with COPD and double-lung transplants reserved for patients with CF or pulmonary fibrosis. Our group reported a retrospective analysis of outcomes after lung transplantation in patients with COPD.[13] In contrast to earlier reports, the morbidity and mortality were comparable for the two groups with an overall hospital mortality of 6.2%. There were no differences in hospital stay, ICU stay, or duration of mechanical ventilation. There was, however, a difference in long-term survival as the 5-year survival of the bilateral transplant recipients was 53%; whereas the survival of the single-lung recipients was 41%. Reports based on the ISHLT database had similar findings, but neither analyses adjusted for factors that might bias such a result, such as the indication for lung transplantation.[14,15] For example, patients receiving double-lung transplants may be more likely to have COPD, which has a significantly better survival.

COMPLICATIONS
Primary Graft Dysfunction

The most feared early complication following lung transplantation is primary graft dysfunction (PGD) which occurs in 11% to 60% of recipients depending on the definition used. PGD clinically, radiographically, and histologically resembles ARDS, but no clear etiology or treatment strategy beyond supportive care has become evident. A recent review of the experience at the author's institution found that the incidence of PGD was approximately 23%, with little difference between the pediatric and adult populations.[16] The indication for lung transplant has some impact on the incidence of PGD where patients with COPD are relatively spared from this condition (18.5%) compared to patients with PPH (29.9%). In this same study, the ischemic time of the lung grafts

developing PGD was slightly longer than grafts that did not develop PGD (290 min ± 86 versus 274 min ± 70), but this did reach statistical significance and appears to have a very minimal causative role. Others have found that lungs obtained from marginal donors were at increased risk for PGD, but these findings were inconsistent among other studies.[17] The only factors consistently associated with PGD development are a recipient history of PPH and a modified reperfusion scheme. Experience at the University of California Los Angeles with a modified preservation solution may also decrease PGD.[18]

PGD heavily impacts short-term outcomes after transplantation, but its influence on long-term survival and the association with BOS are less clear. PGD increases early mortality and ICU and hospital length of stay. Fischer and colleagues found that the survival of patients who survive to hospital discharge following the development of PGD was unchanged relative to patients without PGD, and that the higher overall mortality rate in the PGD cohort was almost entirely attributable to early deaths.[19,20] Conversely, the authors' experience has shown trends toward the development of chronic rejection at an earlier time in patients that experienced PGD when compared to patients that did not.[16,21] More recently, Whitson and colleagues found that freedom from BOS was greater in patients not affected by PGD. These subjects also had higher survival rates at 5 and 10 years. Furthermore, correlations were found between PGD severity and worse long-term outcomes.

Management of PGD remains purely supportive without any known effective treatment strategy to reduce the inflammatory insult. Supplementary oxygen and diuresis are frequently utilized with mechanical ventilation, if necessary. Since reperfusion injury and PGD are often associated with increased pulmonary artery pressures, inhaled nitric oxide has been utilized to mitigate lung injury, although conflicting data exist relating to its efficacy.[17] Theoretically, inhaled nitric oxide replenishes nitric oxide stores in the transplanted lung grafts and helps alleviate ventilation perfusion mismatches. In addition, nitric oxide may diminish inflammatory cytokines released by resident alveolar macrophages.

Less severe forms of the PGD can be treated with supplemental oxygen or mechanical ventilation. The most extreme cases of PGD may require the institution of ECMO in order for the patient to survive. The greatest success of ECMO is typically found in patients requiring ECMO within the first 24 hours after transplantation and in those successfully weaned from ECMO within 48 hours of its institution.[22,23] ECMO may help the lungs recover by decreasing PVR, improve oxygenation, and support the patient through a critical point in their postoperative care.[24] The need for postoperative ECMO conveys a 62% in-hospital mortality rate with multisystem organ failure contributing to the greatest number of deaths in this patient population.[19]

When added to high-potassium preservation solutions, prostaglandin E (PGE) has shown beneficial effects in reducing the occurrence of PGD. However, this beneficial effect has not been observed when lungs are preserved with low-potassium dextran solutions which are currently the most common solution used. PGE may be most beneficial when administered to the transplanted lungs at the time of reperfusion, when the lungs were preserved with a low-potassium solution by altering the inflammatory cytokines released in an animal model.[25]

The impact of PGD on patient outcomes is tremendous. The early mortality rate for patients with PGD is 28.8% compared to 4.2% for patients without PGD. In fact, the phenomenon of PGD was responsible for more early deaths following transplantation than all other perioperative complications combined. PGD also contributes heavily to an increased hospital and ICU length of stay and overall cost of the procedure. Another controversial issue with patients who experience PGD is the option for acute retransplantation, which has an expected high rate of morbidity and mortality for the patient with graft dysfunction and also implications for the survival of patients on the waiting list. In addition, numerous studies have found that the presence of PGD is associated with earlier development of bronchiolitis obliterans and decreased survival (**Figs. 3 and 4**).[16,20,26,27] Patients with the most severe extent of PGD that required ECMO within the first 48 hours after surgery had an early mortality rate of 62%.

Bronchiolitis Obliterans Syndrome

PGD represents the major source of morbidity and mortality in the early post-transplant period, whereas, the development of BOS is the major contributor to long-term morbidity and death. Approximately one half of both pediatric and adult transplanted patients develop BOS within 5 years of transplantation.[16] The etiology of BOS has not been completely elucidated, but it is generally understood to represent chronic rejection. Factors associated with BOS included a history of perioperative PGD, and more recently, gastric reflux and aspiration have been implicated. Neither treating patients with induction immunosuppressive

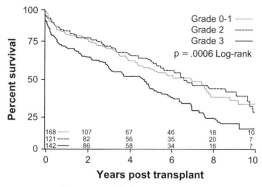

Fig. 3. Overall survival of all 448 lung transplant recipients, grouped by worst PGD grade within the first 48 hours post-transplant [T(0–48)]. Number at risk shown above the x-axis. (*From* Whitson BA, Prekker ME, Herrington TPM, et al. Primary graft dysfunction and long-term pulmonary function after lung transplantation. J Heart Lung Transplant 2007;26:1006; with permission.)

therapy nor differing combinations of calcineurin inhibitors (cyclosporine or tacrolimus) and purine synthesis inhibitors (imuran and mycophenolate) appear to influence the overall incidence or timing of BOS onset.[1] Several proposed therapies for BOS including azithromycin and total lymphoid irradiation reportedly stabilize lung function. In addition, statins and inhaled cyclosporine potentially reduce the incidence of BOS.

Recently, the role for acid and nonacid reflux have been reported.[28] Forty-eight percent of patients had evidence of reflux, half of which were exclusively nonacid reflux as the result of the use of proton pump inhibitors. Not surprisingly, neither pepsin nor bile acids were reduced by proton pump inhibitors. Perhaps bile acids within the airways may play a more causative role in BOS than acid reflux because the presence of bile acids correlated more closely with BOS than either pepsin or acid reflux.[28] With growing evidence that gastric reflux contributes significantly to BOS in transplanted lungs, the role for surgical treatment of GERD may be indicated in this patient population.

Newer methodologies are emerging for early detection of BOS. The exhaled endogenous biomarkers for airway inflammation, nitric oxide, and carbon monoxide have been investigated for early detection of BOS in a time frame that precedes evidence of declining pulmonary function. Others have used inhaled helium washout curves and ^{3}He in conjunction with functional MRI to evaluate ventilation heterogeneity. The ultimate goal of these newer studies is to diagnose BOS at an earlier point in the course of the disease

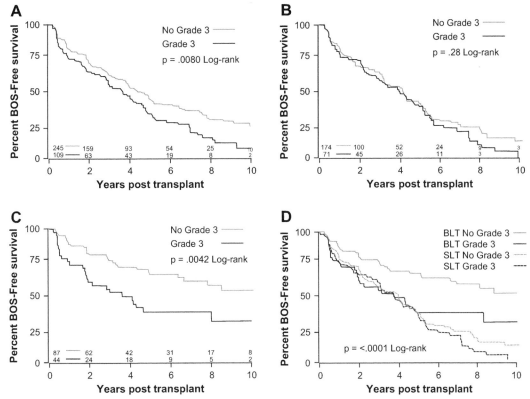

Fig. 4. BOS-free patient survival rates of 90-day survivors, grouped by the occurrence or nonoccurrence of Grade 3 PGD in the first 48 hours post-transplant [T(0–48)], of: (*A*) all 90-day survivors; (*B*) single-lung transplant (SLT); (*C*) BLT; and (*D*) both SLT and BLT recipients. Number at risk shown above the x-axis. (*From* Whitson BA, Prekker ME, Herrington TPM, et al. Primary graft dysfunction and long-term pulmonary function after lung transplantation. J Heart Lung Transplant 2007;26(10):1008; with permission.)

to facilitate earlier treatments. Unfortunately, there are no current treatment strategies available that have gained general acceptance among transplant centers. BOS remains a recalcitrant progressive disease process contributing greatly to long-term pulmonary graft failure and death among lung transplant recipients.

Airway Complications

Postoperative airway anastomotic strictures occur in 7% to 15% of all patients with lung transplants, contributing to the long-term morbidity and reduced pulmonary function. The authors' experience has found an airway complication rate of 9.3% in the adult population over the past decade, but the incidence appears to be declining.[16] Patients that develop airway strictures are not at risk for earlier death relative to patients without strictures. However, repetitive bronchoscopies are typically necessary to palliate this situation and detract from the patient's quality of life. Anastomotic strictures are typically identified within

2 to 6 months of the operation, and their presence correlates with moderate to severe airway ischemia in the immediate postoperative period.[29] Multiple modalities have been utilized to address this issue including laser, brachytherapy, endoscopic stenting, and balloon dilatation, although none of these strategies are completely satisfactory.

When managed initially with balloon dilation, an immediate increase in airway diameter was found in the vast majority of patients, leading to both symptomatic and objective improvements for the majority of patients.[29] Long-term success with balloon dilatation alone was found in approximately one half of the patients, others required subsequent treatments including airway stenting.[29,30] Silicone stents and covered self-expanding metal stents were the earliest devices utilized for this indication, but they are troubled with migration, mucus plugging, and the development of granulation tissue after 3 to 4 months. The rates of these complications improved following the introduction of the nitinol self-expanding metal stents.[31] In a small series of patients treated with nitinol stents, airway patency without significant stenosis persisted without recurrent stenosis for at least a year. Larger studies will be required to confirm the efficacy of currently available airway devices and products still in development. More recently, radiation has also been introduced as a treatment modality to control the rate of restructuring.[32]

SUMMARY

Lung transplantation in the modern era remains an evolving field and a viable option for patients suffering from end-stage emphysema. Recent modifications for recipient prioritization has resulted in a modest decrease in the number of patients with emphysema receiving transplants. More time will be required to determine what impact, if any, these modifications will have on the overall survival of patients with end-stage emphysema. Ongoing research will address persistent issues with lung transplantation, most notably, primary graft dysfunction and chronic BOS.

REFERENCES

1. Trulock EP, Christie JD, Edwards LB, et al. Registry of the International Society for Heart and Lung Transplantation: twenty-fourth official lung and heart-lung transplantation report- 2007. J Heart Lung Transplant 2007;26:782–95.
2. McCue JD, Mooney J, Quail J, et al. Ninety-day mortality and major complications are not affected by use of lung allocation score. J Heart Lung Transplant 2008;27:192–6.
3. Kozower BD, Meyers BF, Smith MA, et al. The impact of the lung allocation score on short-term transplantation outcomes: a multicenter study. J Thorac Cardiovasc Surg 2008;135:166–71.
4. Detterbeck FC, Egan JJ, Mill MR. Lung transplantation after previous thoracic surgical procedures. Ann Thorac Surg 1995;60:139–43.
5. Park S, Nguyen D, Savik K, et al. Pre-transplant corticosteroid use and outcome in lung transplantation. J Heart Lung Transplant 2000;21:304–9.
6. Meyers BF, Lynch JP, Battafarano RJ, et al. Lung transplantation is warranted for stable ventilator dependent recipients. Ann Thorac Surg 2000;70:1675–8.
7. Davis SQ, Garrity ER Jr. Organ allocation in lung transplant. Chest 2007;132:1646–51.
8. UNOS website. Available at: www.unos.org/resources/frm_LAS_Calculator.asp. Accessed April 4, 2009.
9. Lingaraju R, Blumenthal NP, Kotloff M, et al. Effects of lung allocation score on waiting list rankings and transplant procedures. J Heart Lung Transplant 2006;25:1167–70.
10. Gaissert HA, Trulock EP, Cooper JD, et al. Comparison of early functional results after volume reduction or lung transplantation for chronic obstructive pulmonary disease. J Thorac Cardiovasc Surg 1996;111:293–5.
11. Hosenpud JD, Bennett LE, Keck BM, et al. Effect of diagnosis on survival benefit of lung transplantation for end-stage lung disease. Lancet 1998;351:24–7.
12. DeMeester J, Smits JMA, Persijn GG, et al. Listing for lung transplantation: life expectancy and transplant effect, stratified by type of end-stage lung disease, the Eurotransplant experience. J Heart Lung Transplant 2001;20:518–24.
13. Sundaresan RS, Shiraishi Y, Trulock EP, et al. Single or bilateral lung transplantation for emphysema? J Thorac Cardiovasc Surg 1996;112:1485–94.
14. Meyer DM, Bennett LE, Novick RJ, et al. Single vs. bilateral, sequential lung transplantation for end-stage emphysema: influence of recipient age on survival and secondary end-points. J Heart Lung Transplant 2001;20:935–41.
15. Thabut G, Christie JD, Ravaud P, et al. Survival after bilateral versus single lung transplantation for patients with chronic obstructive pulmonary disease: a retrospective analysis of registry data. Lancet 2008;371:744–51.
16. Meyers BF, de la Morena M, Sweet SC, et al. Primary graft dysfunction and other selected complications of lung transplantation: a single-center experience of 983 patients. J Thorac Cardiovasc Surg 2005;129:1421–9.
17. Carter YM, Davis RD. Primary graft dysfunction in lung transplantation. Semin Respir Crit Care Med 2006;27:5014–56.
18. Schnickel GT, Ross DJ, Beygui R. Modified reperfusion in clinical lung transplantation: the result of 100 consecutive cases. J Thorac Cardiovasc Surg 2006;131:218–23.
19. Fischer AJ, Wardle J, Dark JH, et al. Nonimmune acute graft injury after lung transplantation and the risk of subsequent bronchiolitis obliterans syndrome (BOS). J Heart Lung Transplant 2002;21:1206–12.
20. Fiser SM, Tribble CG, Long SM, et al. Ischemia-reperfusion injury after lung transplantation increases risk of late bronchiolitis obliterans syndrome. Ann Thorac Surg 2002;73:1041–8.
21. Bharat A, Narayanan K, Street T, et al. Early post-transplant inflammation promotes the development of alloimmunity and chronic human lung allograft rejection. Transplantation 2007;83:150–8.
22. Meyers BF, Sundt TM III, Henry S, et al. Selective use of extracorporeal membrane oxygenation is warranted after lung transplantation. J Thorac Cardiovasc Surg 2000;120:20–6.

23. Nguyen DQ, Kullick DM, Bolman RM 3rd, et al. Temporary ECMO support following lung and heart-lung transplantation. J Heart Lung Transplant 2000;19:313–6.

24. Hartwig MG, Appel JZ, Cantu E. Improved results treating lung allograft failure with venovenous extracorporal membrane oxygenation. Ann Thorac Surg 2005;80:1872–80.

25. de Perrot M, Liu M, Jin R, et al. Prostaglandin protects lung transplants for ischemia-reperfusion injury: a shift from pro- to anti-inflammatory cytokines. Transplantation 2001;72:1505–12.

26. Burton CM, Iversen M, Milman N, et al. Outcome of lung transplanted patients with primary graft dysfunction. Eur J Cardiothorac Surg 2007;31:75–82.

27. Whitson BA, Prekker ME, Herrington CS, et al. Primary graft dysfunction and long-term pulmonary function after lung transplantation. J Heart Lung Transplant 2007;26:1004–11.

28. Blondeau K, Mertens V, Vanaudenaerde BA, et al. Acid, nonacid GER and gastric aspiration in lung transplant patients with or without chronic rejection. Eur Respir J 2008;31:707–13.

29. DeGracia J, Culebras M, Alvarez A, et al. Bronchoscopic balloon dilation in the management of bronchial stenosis following lung transplantation. Respir Med 2007;101:27–33.

30. Ferretti G, Jouvan FB, Thony F, et al. Benign noninflammatory bronchial stenosis: treatment with balloon dilation. Radiology 1995;196:831–4.

31. Chhajed PN, Malouf MA, Tamm M, et al. Ultraflex stents for the management of airway complications in lung transplant recipients. Respirology 2003;8:59–64.

32. Tendulkar RD, Fleming PA, Reddy CA, et al. High-dose endobronchial brachytherapy for recurrent airway obstruction from hyperplastic granulation tissue. Int J Radiat Oncol Biol Phys 2008;70:701–6.

Index

Note: Page numbers of article titles are in **boldface** type.

A

A1AD. See *Alpha-1 antitrypsin deficiency.*

Air leaks
  and chronic obstructive pulmonary disease, 224
  and emphysema, 223–230
  incidence of, 224
  intraoperative management of, 224–226
  management following lung volume reduction surgery, 227–229
  management of prolonged, 229–230
  postoperative management of, 226–227
  prevention of, 224–225
  repair of, 225–226
  risk factors for, 224

Airway bypass
  concept and evaluation of, 240–241
  laboratory studies evaluating the safety and feasibility of, 241–242
  with paclitaxel-eluting stents, 242
  steps in, 244

Airway bypass treatment of severe homogenous emphysema: taking advantage of collateral ventilation, **239–245**

Alpha-1 antitrypsin deficiency
  and chronic obstructive pulmonary disease, 201–207
  and emphysema, 151–152, 201, 207
  incidence and pathophysiology of, 201–202
  and lung transplantation, 203
  and lung volume reduction surgery, 201–207
  presentation and medical therapy for, 202–203
  and smoking, 202

B

Biomass fuels
  and emphysema, 152–153

BOS. See *Bronchiolitis obliterans syndrome.*

Bronchiolitis obliterans syndrome
  and lung transplantation, 280–281

Bronchopulmonary dysplasia
  and emphysema, 152

C

Chronic obstructive pulmonary disease, 149–156
  and air leaks, 224
  and alpha-1 antitrypsin deficiency, 201–207
  and lung transplantation, 275–279

and lung volume reduction surgery in lung cancer patients, 214

and secondary spontaneous pneumothorax, 233–237

staging of, 151, 154

Coal miners
  emphysema in, 152

Collateral ventilation
  and emphysema, 256
  and homogeneous emphysema, 239–244

Combined cardiac and lung volume reduction surgery, **217–221**
  advantages of, 220
  and coronary artery disease, 217–221
  literature review, 217

Computed tomography
  and emphysema, 159–165

Concomitant lung cancer resection and lung volume reduction surgery, **209–216**

COPD. See *Chronic obstructive pulmonary disease.*

Coronary artery disease
  and combined cardiac and lung volume reduction surgery, 217–221

D

Decision making in the management of secondary spontaneous pneumothorax in patients with severe emphysema, **233–238**

DNDD. See *Donations after neurologic determination of death.*

Donations after neurologic determination of death
  and lung transplantation, 261–264, 267

Donor criteria
  extension of, 264–266

Dyspnea
  and homogeneous emphysema, 196

E

EASE trial. See *Exhale Airway Stents for Emphysema trial.*

EBV. See *Endobronchial valves.*

Emphysema
  acute exacerbations of, 155
  and air leaks, 223–230
  and airway anatomy, variance, and safety score, 163–164
  and alpha-1 antitrypsin deficiency, 151–152, 201–207

doi:10.1016/S1547-4127(09)00026-7

thoracic.theclinics.com

M

N

Printed and bound by CPI Group (UK) Ltd, Croydon, CR0 4YY

03/10/2024

01040353-0015